Physician Burnout

Physician Burnout: How to Rise Above a Broken Healthcare System as a Practicing Clinician is a comprehensive self-help guide that provides practical strategies based on groundbreaking research to help physicians overcome burnout.

Written by a board-certified psychiatrist who provides mental healthcare to physicians, this book is rich in pragmatic, evidence-based strategies to help the reader be better equipped to navigate the daily rigors of practicing medicine. It contains countless clinical examples that illustrate how to overcome burnout and rise above the ever-complex and fragmented landscape of the U.S. healthcare system.

In addition, this book examines how the healthcare system contributes to physician suffering and provides recommendations for improving the culture of medicine.

This book is an essential read for physicians and trainees suffering from burnout as well as anyone who cares about the future of medicine.

Dimitrios Tsatiris, M.D., is a practicing board-certified psychiatrist, TEDx speaker and writer for *Psychology Today*. He is a leading voice at the intersection of mental health and achievement whose mission is to help professionals live their best lives by developing a healthy relationship with achievement.

"Dr. Tsatiris provides the reader with a number of evidence-based strategies to overcome burnout by blending the latest literature with his clinical experience working directly with physicians. The result is an excellent resource for any physician struggling with burnout and for institutions looking to eradicate it."

Beth Frates, M.D., *associate professor, Harvard Medical School,*
president, American College of Lifestyle Medicine

"With his book, Dr. Tsatiris is opening the door to real action and evidence-based approaches that address the bleak landscape of physician burnout. This book should be sent to every medical student upon acceptance to medical school."

Wolfgang Gilliar, D.O., FAAPMR, *dean and chief academic*
officer at Touro University Nevada College of
Osteopathic Medicine (TUNCOM), in Henderson,
Nevada, international speaker and author of over twenty books

"This book lays out the current problems with our unwell medical culture in an elegant, data-driven manner. Physicians will see themselves in many of the outlined scenarios. Drawn from his extensive experience as a psychiatrist, Dr. Tsatiris provides self-driven and systems-driven solutions to deal with the epidemic of burnout."

Dawn L Baker, M.D., M.S., *physician, coach, author of*
Lean Out: A Professional Woman's Guide to
Finding Authentic Work-Life Balance,
and host of the Lean Out *Podcast*

"This book is a must-read for healthcare professionals and leaders navigating the intense pressures of modern medicine. It offers a compassionate and honest look at physician burnout – acknowledging the feelings of betrayal, personal doubts, and the systemic issues that push us beyond our sustainable limits. With practical strategies for both personal and institutional well-being, it will resonate with anyone who cares about the health of our healers and the future of medicine."

Al'ai Alvarez, M.D., *clinical associate professor and*
director of Well-Being at Stanford Emergency Medicine,
nationally recognized for his leadership in
physician wellness and DEI initiatives

Physician Burnout

How to Rise Above a Broken
Healthcare System as a Practicing
Clinician

Dimitrios Tsatiris

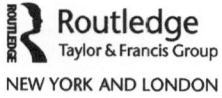
Routledge
Taylor & Francis Group

NEW YORK AND LONDON

Contents

Acknowledgments

This book would not be possible without the physicians I have had the opportunity to serve. Working directly with them has been a privilege. I am grateful for every physician who has trusted me with their care.

I also want to thank Dr. Joseph Varley and Dr. Robert McGregor who spearheaded the creation of the Akron Physician Wellness Initiative (APWI). In addition, I want to thank Dr. Christina Rowan, the clinical director of APWI. Her support in coordinating care, promoting physician wellness and writing this book has been invaluable.

Furthermore, I would like to thank Sarah Rae and Eleanor Broadhurst, editors at Routledge/Taylor & Francis Group for their support, help and guidance on this project.

Most importantly, I want to thank my wife, Deena, and two children, Maria and Michael, who cheered me on as I worked on this project. This book would not have come to life without their love, understanding and support.

Introduction

Remember Who You Are

You are resilient.

If there is only one thing you take from this book, let it be this.

You may not feel resilient at this moment. You might feel dejected because medicine has not turned into the career you had envisioned. Becoming a physician was a calling to care for people and help them live their best lives. Unfortunately, you do not feel like you are fulfilling this mission. Instead, you feel like a cog in a bureaucratic machine that makes it impossible to actually care for patients.

Your feelings are valid and understandable. Becoming a physician was no easy feat. During college, you spent countless hours studying while simultaneously building an impressive resume of prestigious awards, research projects and volunteer opportunities to meet the rigorous standards of getting into medical school. While many of your classmates spent their weekends socializing, you volunteered at the local hospital or studied for the MCAT. Many aspired to get into medical school. However, you had the dedication and perseverance to make your dream a reality.

The stakes only intensified in medical school. You spent countless hours in a cold, dark anatomy lab carefully dissecting every muscle on a human cadaver to learn its origin, insertion and innervation. You spent entire days at your school's library memorizing the steps of the Krebs cycle and the pharmacokinetics of different drugs. In the meantime, peers who had pursued careers outside medicine were wrapping up their studies and getting a head start in life.

The sacrifices only continued in residency where you missed countless family gatherings because you had to work night shifts, weekends and holidays. Despite the grueling workload, you somehow found time to study for intense board exams that spanned 16 hours over two days. The emotional toll from these sacrifices was further exacerbated by harsh, and often unfair, criticisms from attending physicians and senior residents. Even though you were learning on the job, their callous comments made

DOI: 10.4324/9781003473923-1

you feel like an imposter and question whether you had what it takes to become a physician.

You put your entire life on hold to become a physician. Finding a life partner was difficult because you devoted your time and energy to medicine. You delayed starting a family or buying a house because you did not know where your career would take you. You also took on significant student loans which ballooned by the end of your medical training. Coupled with the delay in your earning years, they made it exponentially harder to find your footing outside medicine.

The majority of people are not willing or able to endure such sacrifices. Your studies after college included four years of medical school, 3–7 years of residency training and an additional year or two of fellowship training. There were many times you felt homesick because you had to leave behind loved ones and travel to different parts of the country to complete these studies. You endured tremendous hardships to become a physician.

The sacrifices have only continued after your medical training. As an attending physician, you have felt the pressure of making urgent medical decisions with a patient's life on the line. You have stayed up all night worrying about your patients as you wondered whether you made the right call. After all, medical knowledge has its limits, beyond which, clinical decisions are judgment calls that come with inherent uncertainty.

You have a front row seat to human suffering. You have witnessed traumatic events that you would have never imagined if you had not become a physician. You have treated people with gruesome injuries from motor vehicle accidents and acts of violence. You have also helped patients who have confided personal stories of emotional and sexual abuse. These experiences haunt you because they are a stark reminder of the fragility and finality that define the human condition.

You have also felt the heartache of losing a patient and the pain of consoling their family. Every loss leaves behind a wound that accompanies you for the rest of your life. The long, lonely walk down the cold hospital corridor to inform family members that their loved one did not survive does not get any easier after all these years.

It took great sacrifices to become a physician. The same holds true for being a physician. Yet, you continue to show up and do your best to serve the next person who needs your help despite how you feel. Your ability to endure hardship and continue to show up for others is undeniable proof of your resilience.

Not that resilience is a panacea against burnout. According to a cross-sectional study of over 5,400 respondents, even the most resilient physicians suffer from high rates of burnout (1). Suffering from burnout is not a resilience issue. You are plenty resilient. Anyone who gives you a wellness lecture on how to be more resilient knows nothing about the sacrifices you have endured or the daily challenges you face. Being a physician is hard. You have a front row seat to human suffering and carry the heavy responsibility of healing those who are sick, ill and hurt. Even if you practiced medicine in ideal settings, it takes tremendous strength to show up while being exposed to the fears, concerns and traumatic experiences of your patients.

Of course, you do not have the luxury of practicing medicine in ideal settings. Far from it. Countless systemic factors have contributed to your burnout because they interfere with your ability to serve patients. Increased administrative, clinical and documentation requirements, a loss of clinical autonomy and authority, denials of care from insurance companies, mounting educational debt, persisting gender and racial inequalities and a fear of being sued stretch you beyond your limits.

The corporatization of healthcare only intensifies the problem. By adopting business metrics to maximize revenue, hospital administrators put you in an impossible moral conundrum. Conforming to their demands of meeting productivity benchmarks, which prioritize profitability, further interferes with your ability to care for patients.

Wendy Dean M.D. uses the term moral injury to describe the dilemma of simultaneously knowing what care is best for patients but being unable to provide it due to barriers that are beyond your control (2). The term emphasizes that you are part of a fragmented healthcare system that interferes with your ability to honor the oath of always putting the patient first. Altruism is associated with worse mental health outcomes when altruistic norms exist but the altruistic behavior cannot occur (3). Unfortunately, this is a common occurrence in medicine.

There is debate about whether burnout or moral injury is the more appropriate term to describe the suffering physicians are going through. Some say the term burnout implies that physicians are responsible for their suffering. I disagree with this interpretation of the term. Physicians are suffering from burnout because of systemic factors that are beyond their control and morally injure them. From this lens, both terms are accurate descriptors of the problem plaguing medicine. They are not mutually exclusive.

As physicians, we have unique traits that helped us endure the long, arduous journey of medical training. In general, we are altruistic, achievement-oriented perfectionists who do not cope well with failure. When someone assigns us a goal, we move heaven and earth to achieve it. We would rather skip sleep, meals and other basic needs than fall below the mark. Though these traits ensure we always put the patient first, they also make us prone to exploitation. The healthcare system is aware of our tendencies and uses them to its advantage, playing a significant role in physician burnout.

What is Burnout?

Burnout was first described by German-born psychologist Herbert Freudenberger. It is a syndrome consisting of three symptoms. The first is emotional exhaustion. A classic example of emotional exhaustion is feeling depleted at work, even though you just came back from vacation. The second is depersonalization which is feeling detached from your work, colleagues and patients. This can manifest as a lack of empathy for your patients or feeling increasingly cynical of colleagues. In many ways, depersonalization is an inability to embrace the humanity in others. The final symptom is having a reduced sense of personal achievement because you believe your career lacks purpose and meaning. When you consider the impact of these symptoms, it is not surprising that burned out physicians contemplate leaving clinical medicine.

Although burnout shares clinical features with depression such as fatigue and low motivation, they are two different constructs. Burnout is more context specific and prevalent in occupations that are emotionally taxing such as healthcare providers, social workers and teachers. On the other hand, depression is more pervasive and expands beyond one's occupation. Though different, each variable can serve as a risk factor for the other. Suffering from burnout makes you more vulnerable to depression and vice versa (4).

If you are suffering from burnout, recognize you are not alone. A 2021 survey showed that nearly 63% of U.S. physicians suffer from burnout. It also showed that burnout had increased compared to the prior year (5). I share this data not to minimize or trivialize your suffering. Rather, I want to highlight that burnout is widespread because systemic factors are having a negative impact on the majority of physicians, including you.

The Cost of Burnout

Burnout does not only have a negative impact on your mental health. It is also a significant predictor for a host of physical health conditions including coronary heart disease, type II diabetes, prolonged fatigue, headaches and mortality below the age of 45 (6). Left untamed, burnout can compromise the quality and length of your life.

Furthermore, burnout can negatively impact your relationship with loved ones. According to a Medscape survey of over 9,100 physicians, 65% of respondents believed that burnout had a negative impact on their relationships (7). This figure is not surprising when you consider that burnout is associated with feeling detached and emotionally depleted. It is difficult to connect with loved ones when you feel this way.

Moreover, burnout can endanger patient care. A survey of nearly 6,700 U.S. physicians found that those who had reported medical errors were more likely to have symptoms of burnout (8). This association is evidence that improving physician well-being is an important intervention to enhance patient safety.

In a desperate effort to survive the devastating effects of burnout and preserve their careers, physicians often reduce their working hours. A longitudinal study of physicians found that every 1-point increase on a 7-point emotional exhaustion scale correlated with a higher likelihood of reducing their working hours (9). Though understandable, this trend is likely to exacerbate the physician shortage plaguing the U.S. healthcare system. According to the Association of American Medical Colleges, the United States could see an estimated shortage ranging between 37,800 and 124,000 physicians by 2034, with shortages in both primary and specialty care (10). Having physicians work fewer hours or retire early due to burnout will only make it harder for patients to access the healthcare they desperately need.

Solutions

Considering the enormous cost of burnout on physicians, patients and the entire healthcare system, addressing the problem is imperative. There are two types of solutions. The first involves a top-down approach in which hospital leadership, insurance companies, the pharmaceutical industry and governing bodies implement policies to address the systemic factors plaguing medicine. Such changes would eventually trickle down to physicians working in the trenches and improve their daily work experience. The second type involves a bottom-top approach in which you employ individual strategies to be better equipped to navigate the systemic factors contributing to burnout.

Ideally, a combination of both types of solutions is employed to eradicate burnout. A systematic review and meta-analysis showed that both individual-focused and structural strategies can reduce burnout among physicians (11). Another meta-analysis showed that organization-driven interventions were more effective in reducing burnout compared to physician-directed interventions (12).

Though essential to eradicate burnout, there are fundamental limitations to relying exclusively on a top-down approach. The first is that such an approach is beyond your sphere of control. Waiting for key players of the healthcare system, who are removed from the realities of day-to-day clinical practice, to respond to your needs in a timely and effective manner is a strategy that is highly unlikely to yield the meaningful change you desperately need .

A look at the landscape of the healthcare system supports my position. The U.S. spends more on healthcare than other high-income nations. Yet, this spending has not translated to better quality of care as the U.S. has the lowest life expectancy and highest suicide rates of the group (13). In addition, the U.S. spends more on administrative expenses than other nations. These expenses account for approximately 15% to 25% of total healthcare spending, which is three times the amount spent on cancer care (14). A review published in *JAMA* estimated the cost of waste to range between $760 billion and $935 billion, which represents almost 25% of total healthcare spending (15). These dismal results highlight the inefficiencies of an inflated system that is unable to address the problems plaguing it. When you consider these inefficiencies, why would you hold out hope that this bloated and fragmented system will evolve into a more organized, efficient and humane establishment that prioritizes patient care and physician wellness?

No, you cannot blindly trust the system. This is why I want to empower you with a number of evidence-based strategies to be best equipped to navigate the current landscape. Focusing on a bottom-top approach helps you be proactive and have more agency in your personal and professional life. Such an approach does not absolve hospitals, governing bodies and other involved parties of their responsibility to address the systemic factors contributing to physician burnout and compromising patient care. These systemic factors are the primary driving force behind the burnout epidemic because they hinder your ability to best care for patients. The healthcare system needs to prioritize patient care by addressing these factors.

In the meantime, you need to embrace a bottom-top approach. This does not mean that suffering from burnout is your fault. You are not to blame for the systemic factors plaguing clinical medicine. You are suffering from burnout because of things that have happened to you, not because of you. However, you are responsible for responding to the difficult hand you have been dealt in a healthy manner. You cannot relinquish this responsibility. Your loved ones, patients and colleagues are counting on you to rise above a broken healthcare system by reclaiming the strengths, skills and resilience that have helped you overcome challenges throughout your life.

There is a difference between being at fault compared to being responsible for something. Fault refers to the past tense and things that have previously transpired outside your control. Responsibility refers to the "here and now" and highlights actions you need to take within your sphere of control. For example, you are not at fault if a patient makes poor lifestyle choices that jeopardize their health such as misuse alcohol or illicit drugs. However, you are responsible for trying to help them when they show up at your office.

Likewise, you are not at fault for the systemic factors plaguing medicine and contributing to your emotional difficulties. However, you are responsible for responding to these factors in a way that minimizes their impact on your health, relationship with loved ones, and patients. Relinquishing this responsibility only exacerbates a bad situation.

Embracing a bottom-top approach highlights the psychological concept of radical acceptance. To radically accept something does not mean you are ok with what is transpiring. The healthcare system is broken and radical action is necessary to address the inefficiencies compromising patient care.

On the contrary, the intent of radical acceptance is to help you stay grounded within your sphere of control. Focusing on everything that is outside your control is a recipe for feeling helpless and powerless. This only makes you more vulnerable to exploitation by systemic factors.

Consistently taking action within your sphere of control leads to an important insight. You have more influence, resilience and options than you realize. You can advocate for yourself and your patients despite systemic forces wanting you to stay silent. You are a competent physician who is having a positive impact on the life of many people regardless of calculated attempts to devalue your role as a physician. You are plenty busy regardless of persistent demands from hospital administrators to work harder to generate more RVUs. Regardless of how they try to make you feel, they can never strip you of your clinical expertise or experience. You are the same resilient person who overcame a mountain of hardships to become a physician. Tapping into your innate resilience will help you rise above the systemic factors plaguing medicine and inspire other struggling colleagues to follow your lead.

I wrote this book with these truths in mind. This book is filled with a number of evidence-based tools that will help you maximize your sphere of control. You can immediately implement them in your life regardless of your specialty, years of clinical experience or setting in which you practice medicine. As a board-certified psychiatrist who has an extensive history of working closely with hundreds of physicians from all walks of life, I have the necessary experience and expertise to help you on your journey.

This book is divided into four parts. The first part, titled *"Know Yourself"*, will take you on a journey of self-discovery. It will help you understand how becoming a physician and practicing medicine have fundamentally changed who you are. The second part, titled *"Know the System"*, describes how the healthcare system has contributed to your burnout. The third part of the book, termed *"A Path to a Better Self"*, is filled with evidence-based tools to help you overcome burnout and find fulfillment in clinical medicine. The last part of the book is titled *"A Path to a Better System"* and describes ways you can positively influence the healthcare system to ensure future generations of physicians experience a better, more humane way of practicing medicine.

Thank you for the opportunity to be of service to you.

References

1. West CP, Dyrbye LN, Sinsky C, et al. Resilience and burnout among physicians and the general US working population. *JAMA Netw Open.* 2020;3(7):e209385. https://doi.org/10.1001/jamanetworkopen.2020.9385
2. Dean W, Talbot S, Dean A. Reframing clinician distress: moral injury not burnout [published correction appears in *Fed Pract.* 2019 Oct;36(10):447]. *Fed Pract.* 2019;36(9):400–402.
3. Feng Y, Zong M, Yang Z, et al. When altruists cannot help: the influence of altruism on the mental health of university students during the COVID-19 pandemic. *Glob Health.* 2020;16:61. https://doi.org/10.1186/s12992-020-00587-y
4. Koutsimani P, Montgomery A, Georganta K. The relationship between burnout, depression, and anxiety: a systematic review and meta-analysis. *Front Psychol.* 2019;10. https://doi.org/10.3389/fpsyg.2019.00284
5. Shanafelt TD, West CP, Dyrbye LN, et al. Changes in burnout and satisfaction with work-life integration in physicians during the first 2 years of the COVID-19 pandemic. *Mayo Clin Proc.* 2022;97(12):2248–2258. https://doi.org/10.1016/j.mayocp.2022.09.002
6. Salvagioni DAJ, Melanda FN, Mesas AE, et al. Physical, psychological and occupational consequences of job burnout: a systematic review of prospective studies. *PloS One.* 2017;12(10):e0185781. https://doi.org/10.1371/journal.pone.0185781
7. Kane L. 'I cry but no one cares': physician burnout and depression report 2023. *Medscape.* January 27, 2023. Accessed October 14, 2023. https://www.medscape.com/slideshow/2023-lifestyle-burnout-6016058
8. Tawfik DS, Profit J, Morgenthaler TI, et al. Physician burnout, well-being, and work unit safety grades in relationship to reported medical errors. *Mayo Clin Proc.* 2018;93(11):1571–1580. https://doi.org/10.1016/j.mayocp.2018.05.014
9. Shanafelt TD, Mungo M, Schmitgen J, et al. Longitudinal study evaluating the association between physician burnout and changes in professional work effort. *Mayo Clin Proc.* 2016;91(4):422–431. https://doi.org/10.1016/j.mayocp.2016.02.001
10. AAMC report reinforces mounting physician shortage. *AAMC.* June 11, 2021. Accessed October 6, 2023. https://www.aamc.org/news/press-releases/aamc-report-reinforces-mounting-physician-shortage
11. West CP, Dyrbye LN, Erwin PJ, Shanafelt TD. Interventions to prevent and reduce physician burnout: a systematic review and meta-analysis. *Lancet.* 2016;388(10057):2272–2281. doi:10.1016/S0140-6736(16)31279-X
12. Panagioti M, Panagopoulou E, Bower P, et al. Controlled interventions to reduce burnout in physicians: a systematic review and meta-analysis. *JAMA Intern Med.* 2017;177(2):195–205. doi:10.1001/jamainternmed.2016.7674
13. Tikkanen R, Abrams MK. U.S. health care from a global perspective, 2019: higher spending, worse outcomes? *Commonwealth Fund.* January, 2020. Accessed February 20, 2024. https://www.commonwealthfund.org/publications/issue-briefs/2020/jan/us-health-care-global-perspective-2019

14. Tollen L, Keating E, Weil A . How administrative spending contributes to excess US health spending. *Health Affairs* blog. February 2020. Accessed February 20, 2024. https://www.healthaffairs.org/do/10.1377/hblog20200218.375060/full/

15. Shrank WH, Rogstad TL, Parekh N. Waste in the US health care system: estimated costs and potential for savings. *JAMA*. 2019;322(15):1501–1509. doi:10.1001/jama.2019.13978

Part 1

Know Yourself

1   You Have Been Betrayed

I want you to go back to the moment you decided to become a physician. Odds are you found your calling at a young age. Perhaps you were inspired by a family member who was a physician and wanted to follow in their footsteps. Or maybe you recognized the importance of health after witnessing a loved one struggle with illness or die young.

Of course, not every physician discovers their calling at a young age. You might have followed a less traditional route and applied to medical school after working for years in a field unrelated to medicine. Interestingly, many of the top performers in my medical school class were older. To this day, I marvel at their ability to excel academically while they balanced family responsibilities in such a rigorous environment. I believe the diversity of their previous life experiences provided them with unique insights and skills that served as a competitive advantage over the typical student entering medical school straight out of college.

Regardless of your path to medicine, you had to consider the tremendous sacrifices required to become a physician. These sacrifices are not for the faint of heart. Taking on hundreds of thousands in student loans to extend your studies by at least seven years after college while missing out on countless family and social events is something that most people would not sign up for. Yet, you decided to delay personal milestones such as buying a house, finding a life partner or starting a family to become a physician. By the time you had completed your training and were finally ready to establish roots, your peers outside medicine had a ten-year head start on you.

What motivated you to pursue a path that most people would pass up? Uncovering the underlying emotional forces that drew you to a career in medicine can help you have a deeper understanding of who you are.

DOI: 10.4324/9781003473923-3

Motivation Theory

A core psychological principle is that unsatisfied needs influence your thoughts and behaviors. This is apparent with your physical needs. Imagine you desperately have to use the bathroom during a mandatory department meeting. Paying attention during the meeting is nearly impossible because you are preoccupied with having to use the bathroom. Every second feels like an eternity as you clench your urethral sphincters tightly for dear life.

Additional physical needs include the need to breathe, sleep, eat and consume water.

Fortunately, we are privileged to meet these needs fairly easily because access to food, water and shelter is readily available. This is when more complex emotional needs come to the forefront. According to the psychologist Abraham Maslow, needs are arranged in a hierarchy with emotional needs becoming more prominent after basic physiologic needs have been met. Examples include the need to feel safe and loved, to have a sense of belonging, feel respected and derive meaning from one's life. At the peak of Maslow's hierarchical pyramid is the need for self-actualization, to use one's abilities and skills to reach their fullest potential (1).

Additional emotional needs have been described by different psychologists studying motivation theory. According to Dr. David McClelland, there are three primary needs that drive human behavior. They include the need to achieve, to accumulate power and to find affiliation. The need to achieve represents a drive for competence as you compete against a task, yourself and others. Those with a high need to achieve pursue goals for the sake of doing so. The need for power represents a drive to influence, and even control others. Those with a high need for power constantly climb the professional ranks in its pursuit. Finally, the need for affiliation manifests as a drive to fit in and please others in interpersonal relationships (2).

Herzberg's two-factor theory applied human motivation theory to the workplace setting. It outlines motivators which promote job satisfaction and hygiene factors which prevent job dissatisfaction. Motivators fulfill intrinsic emotional needs such as the need for recognition, achievement and personal growth. Hygiene factors address extrinsic factors such as pay grade, work culture, working conditions and administrative practices (3).

Emotional Needs

Emotional needs have shaped your behavior since childhood. Consider how the need to achieve has fueled your lifelong drive towards academic excellence. From a young age, you received grades based on your performance on a homework assignment or exam. This measuring system served as both a carrot and stick to earn the highest grade possible. You felt proud of yourself when you received accolades from your parents and teachers for earning high grades. Lower grades were met with disapproval, even harsh criticism, resulting in unpleasant feelings. In response to this combination of positive reinforcement and punishment, you learned to constantly compete against yourself to earn the highest grade possible.

The grading system also reinforced your need to achieve by placing you in an undeclared competition against peers. Being an A student resulted in more recognition and accolades compared to someone with lower grades. It also provided you with unique academic opportunities which further differentiated you from the pack.

Though established early in childhood, emotional needs influence your behaviors throughout adulthood. As an example, medicine has reinforced your need to achieve. During medical school, you competed against yourself to earn the highest grade possible on written or clinical exams. You also worked hard to outperform your peers because your class ranking determined how competitive you were as an applicant for residency programs. This pattern only continued in residency because you had to stand apart from your peers to become chief resident, get into a competitive fellowship program or find a desirable job as an attending physician.

A look at different emotional needs shows how much they influence the way you think and act. The need for connection is the reason you took a leap of faith at some point in your life to pursue a long-term relationship. The need for security is the reason most physicians accept a lower paying job as a hospital employee compared to the potentially more lucrative, but also riskier, option of starting their own private practice. The need to find meaning and purpose is what motivates many of us to become physicians or start families. The need for power and control is what drives some to constantly climb the academic and administrative ranks in order to control those with less power. The need for recognition is why some overextend themselves financially hoping to stand out when they buy a fancy house or car.

Though unnoticed, emotional needs influence even your most subtle daily habits. The need to feel safe is the reason you lock your doors before going to bed or double check the stove to make sure it is turned off on your way out the door. The need for recognition is why some spend countless hours on social media chasing likes and followers. The need to belong is why you stay silent when boundaries are violated at home or work. The risk of compromising a relationship and being cast away can be too much to bear.

We all share the same emotional needs. After all, they are needs, not wants. What differentiates us is the amount of energy, time and effort it takes to satisfy them.

As an example, let's consider the need for connection. You may be a raging introvert, like myself, who relishes alone time. Your ideal weekend may be staying at home, reading books and doing yardwork in silence. Such a weekend would be torture for an extrovert who recharges their batteries by being out and about with friends and family. Extroverts undoubtedly have a greater need for connection as they require more time with a larger number of people to satisfy this need. However, even the most introverted of introverts needs to meaningfully connect with someone, be it a human, pet or plant.

The reason you became a physician was to fulfill different emotional needs. At the top of the list was your need to make a positive difference in the life of others. You were motivated by a pure and selfless zeal to help those suffering from health ailments. Medicine is not just a career. It is a calling to serve others. Your oath to put patients first is the moral compass that guides every clinical decision.

However, altruism is not the only factor that led you to medicine. After all, one can fulfill their altruistic need to serve in a variety of settings. You could have chosen to become a teacher, firefighter, counselor, psychologist, nurse or social worker to serve people. This indicates that a number of other factors influenced you to become a physician. A systematic literature review of cross-sectional studies from different countries identified a number of such motivating factors (4). Since we come from different backgrounds with different upbringings, it would be a gross oversimplification to assign altruism as the only motive that drives someone to become a physician.

Some pursued a career in medicine with the hopes of being recognized as successful. They believed that earning a prestigious title, wearing the white coat and having an office filled with degrees and awards would elevate them in the eyes of others.

Others became physicians to fulfill their need for security. As physicians, we hold stable jobs with relatively healthy incomes. The potential of a financially secure future could have played a role in your decision-making, especially if you came from humble beginnings. However, do not mistaken financial security with becoming wealthy. If wealth accumulation was your primary motive, then medicine was not the best choice. You would have been better served to pursue a career in business rather than delay your earning years by 7–10 years after college while accumulating student loans.

Perhaps becoming a physician was more about fulfilling the dreams of your parents rather than your own. I have worked with physicians who revealed that their parents pushed them from a young age to enter clinical medicine. If this was your case, then your need to please others influenced your career choices.

You might have even pursued clinical medicine because of your high need to achieve. Due to its constantly evolving nature, medicine is appealing to achievement-oriented individuals who are constantly challenging themselves to learn new information. I have even talked to residents who were ready to become attending physicians but chose to extend their training for an extra year and pursue a fellowship even though it did not directly affect their job prospects. It is as if they had been in school for so long that they felt uncomfortable with the idea of not having a teacher to report to.

Before reading any further, take a few minutes to reflect on the underlying emotional forces that influenced you to become a physician. What emotional needs were you hoping to fulfill by becoming a physician?

Affect Forecasting

Regardless of your motive, you decided to pursue a career in medicine by looking into the future. You believed that the sacrifices to become a physician would ultimately be worth it because there would be a reward at the end of your training. The process of trying to predict how future events will make us feel is known as affect forecasting.

Naturally, we pursue paths that we believe will be favorable in some way. In general, we can fairly accurately predict how future events influence the quality of our emotions. For example, you would agree that receiving a check in the mail for $1 million as a gift will elicit more positive feelings compared to receiving a notice that you owe $1 million in unpaid taxes.

However, our crystal ball is cloudy when trying to predict the future and we fall for traps. Let's explore a few of them.

Impact Bias

The first trap is known as the impact bias. Though we can accurately predict the quality of our future emotions, we misjudge their duration and intensity. In particular, we overestimate how much happier we will feel after achieving a particular goal (5).

As an example, consider how you felt after you completed your medical school training. You certainly felt a sense of pride and joy when you received your diploma at graduation. How long did those warm, fuzzy feelings last? Did they even last a few months? Odds are it was early in your residency training when they were replaced by feelings of anxiety and burnout.

The reason we fall for the impact bias is because of our distorted view on achievement. We only focus on the bright side of success such as being recognized for our feats or its financial benefits. However, we ignore the negative aspects of achievement such as being under greater scrutiny or carrying increased responsibilities. The reality is that it is not always sunny with clear blue skies when you successfully make it to the top of your mountain. There will be plenty of overcast days with strong winds and heavy rains.

The impact bias served an important purpose. Idealizing your dreams provided you with the necessary motivation to endure the hardships of your training. The sacrifices of your journey were more palatable because you believed there would be a pot of gold at the end of your odyssey. Holding onto an idealized version of clinical medicine helped you stay the course throughout medical school and residency training.

As an example, it is not uncommon for medical school students to be in denial or ignore how much they owe in student loans. This can serve as a powerful defense mechanism to stay focused on one's goal of graduating medical school. To this day, I vividly remember this process play out a few weeks prior to graduation, when my medical school had arranged for our class to meet with a loan officer. We each received a sealed letter with the remaining balance of our student loans and repayment options. Many classmates broke out into tears after opening their letter. Others looked stunned and in disbelief questioning whether they had received the correct letter. You can escape reality for only so long before it strikes you in the face.

Arrival Fallacy

The other trap when trying to forecast the future is known as the arrival fallacy. This is the process of believing that you will finally be happy when you achieve a future goal such as being accepted into medical school, becoming a physician, getting married, buying your dream house, building a successful practice or making it to retirement. It takes the form of: "I will be happy when I [choose your future goal]."

The problem with this pattern of thinking is that your happiness becomes conditional on achieving an idealized future outcome that may ultimately let you down. This is because any goal you strive towards is skewed by the impact bias. Beware of the destination as it may not turn out as you had imagined it.

The Betrayal

What causes great pain is the realization that medicine has not turned into the career you had imagined. You endured countless hardships believing they would ultimately be worth it. However, you have been betrayed because medicine has not fulfilled any of your emotional needs. Rather, it has been a major source of frustration, angst and disappointment.

You might have entered medicine with the purest intentions of making a positive contribution in the life of others. However, on a daily basis, you encounter systemic barriers that interfere with your ability to provide the best care possible. For example, you might prescribe a medication to address your patient's health concern only to have an insurance company deny coverage because it is not included in their formulary of covered medications. You might want to spend more time with your patients to explore their concerns in greater depth, but have to cut the appointment short due to being overbooked with too many patients. What precious, little time you have with patients is further disrupted by cumbersome documentation requirements which do not enhance patient care. All this, while the fear of litigation constantly hovers in the background and sways you to practice defensive medicine.

You might have thought that earning a medical degree and wearing a white coat would elevate you in the eyes of others. You would be recognized as an expert who worked hard to develop your current clinical knowledge and skills. The truth is there has been a systematic attempt to diminish the value of your medical degree. Insurance companies and hospitals refer to physicians as providers. This term implies you have the same qualifications, training and expertise as advanced practice providers, which is simply not accurate. Lumping you in the same category as everyone else is intended to diminish your authority and autonomy, making you more vulnerable to exploitation.

Pointing out this tactic is not intended to minimize the importance of advanced practice providers who play an essential role in patient care. They are an indispensable part of the healthcare team in every setting. Rather, the intention is to show how systemic factors are eroding the patient-physician relationship. Referring to everyone who delivers care as a provider makes it harder for patients to decipher the qualifications and training of the individual providing their care. This tactic devalues the patient-physician relationship and implies that any provider can substitute the treating physician.

Being a physician no longer carries the same weight in society. The rise of social media has made it easier for people to access and spread health information. Unfortunately, it has also facilitated the spread of medical misinformation by individuals who lack proper training. It feels as if society would rather garner their health information from online influencers with large followings instead of qualified physicians with years of clinical experience. As an example, I had a patient agree with my recommendations on how to treat her anxiety disorder because they were aligned with recommendations from her health coach. Being a board-certified psychiatrist with over a decade of clinical experience was outweighed by a health coach without the same level of education or training.

If you entered medicine seeking financial security, then you may be greatly disappointed. Accumulating an average of $200,000 in medical student loans while delaying your earning years is not a recipe for financial security (6). I have also seen resident physicians struggle to find employment upon graduation. In the past ten years, the number of physicians working as hospital employees has increased, while the number of physicians working in private practice has decreased (7). This trend is an understandable response to financial pressures stemming from reduced Medicare reimbursements, rising operating costs for practices and increased administrative burdens. However, this trend comes at a cost. By relinquishing our leverage to hospitals, physicians are having a harder time finding clinically meaningful work with fair compensation and work-life balance. As a result, many graduating resident physicians are settling for jobs with lower pay, increased work hours and responsibilities not necessarily aligned with their skillset and preferences.

Another concerning trend that makes a career in medicine less financially secure is the dramatic rise in the monetary amounts awarded in malpractice lawsuits. In 2023, there were 57 medical malpractice verdicts of $10 million or more in the United States with more than half reaching at least $25 million. Such verdicts can have lasting effects on future claims by driving up the cost to resolve them (8).

If your need to achieve motivated you to become a physician, then you have been let down. Medicine demands perfection. Even the slightest shortcoming is met with harsh criticism. As a resident, you were constantly under the microscope. Writing even a single, substandard note on the most hectic of call nights would elicit a punitive reaction from your supervising physician. Being a seasoned attending physician has not made you exempt from such a reaction. Even a single negative score on a patient satisfaction survey can elicit an unforgiving response from your employer. Instead of being treated like a competent professional, you feel like an imposter who is not doing an adequate job. The spotlight is on your shortcomings, while there is barely any recognition of your contributions to your patients and hospital system.

Medicine has not turned into the career that you had envisioned. Regardless of your motives, you have been betrayed. You sacrificed your best years to become a physician, only to be saddled with student loans, systemic barriers that interfere with your ability to provide care and a lack of appreciation for your hard work. You are constantly looking over your shoulder fearing the next punishment for failing to meet expectations. What's worse is you feel trapped in medicine. Financial restrictions, family commitments and a lack of cross-training for alternative careers make it difficult to leave medicine. You are carrying a deep wound that leaves you feeling cynical and hopeless about your current state of affairs and future prospects.

In the words of an early-career attending:

> I sacrificed four years of my life to complete medical school. As painful as it was, I stayed the course thinking it would ultimately be worth it. I did not feel an ounce happier in residency. Yet, I endured residency by telling myself that life would be better as an attending. Here I am. I have been wrong and regret my choices.

Many physicians regret their decision to pursue a career in medicine. A 2021 survey of 2,440 physicians showed that only 57.1% of respondents would choose medicine again (9). A poll of over 12,000 physicians on Doximity showed that 60% of them would not want their children to work in medicine (10). Such figures highlight how disillusioned physicians are with the current landscape in healthcare.

Coming to the painful realization that medicine has not come even close to being the career you had envisioned is not intended to send you in despair. Give yourself grace. Your younger self could not have foreseen how things would turn out. Medicine hides its flaws behind a veil and catches all newcomers off guard. They become apparent only after you spend considerable time in medicine to familiarize yourself with its inner workings.

You are not alone. The fact that many physicians are suffering and would not recommend a career in medicine is evidence that you are not the problem. You are not at fault for your suffering, but are responsible for doing your best to navigate the dire situation at hand. Recognizing and accepting that you have been betrayed by medicine is the first step to breaking free from the shackles of burnout.

References

1. Taormina RJ, Gao JH. Maslow and the motivation hierarchy: measuring satisfaction of the needs. *The American Journal of Psychology.* 2013;126(2):155–177. https://doi.org/10.5406/amerjpsyc.126.2.0155   https://www.jstor.org/stable/10.5406/amerjpsyc.126.2.0155
2. McClelland, DC. *The achieving society.* Van Nostrand Company, Inc. 1961. http://doi:10.2307/3111921
3. Herzberg F. *Work and the nature of man.* World Publishing Company. 1966.
4. Goel S, Angeli F, Dhirar N, Singla N, Ruwaard D. What motivates medical students to select medical studies: a systematic literature review. *BMC Med Educ.* 2018 Jan 17;18(1):16. doi:10.1186/s12909-018-1123-4
5. Wilson T, Gilbert D. Affect forecasting. *Advances in Experimental Social Psychology.* 2003;35:345–411.

6. Medical student education: debt, costs, and loan repayment fact card for the class of 2023. *AAMC*. October, 2023. Accessed March 16, 2024. https://store. aamc.org/medical-student-education-debt-costs-and-loan-repayment-fact-card-for-the-class-of-2023.html

7. Landi H. Docs shift to larger, hospital-owned practices to have more negotiation power with payers, AMA analysis finds. *Fierce Healthcare*. July, 2023. Accessed March 16, 2024. https://www.fiercehealthcare.com/providers/docs-shift-larger-hospital-owned-practices-have-more-negotiation-power-payers-ama

8. Gallegos, A. Mega malpractice verdicts against physicians on the rise. *Medscape Medical News*. February, 2024. Accessed March 20, 2024. https://www.medscape.com/viewarticle/mega-malpractice-verdicts-against-physicians-rise-2024a10002bz#:~:text=In%202023%2C%20there%20were%2057,in%202022%2C%20TransRe%20research%20found.

9. Shanafelt TD, West CP, Dyrbye LN, et al. Changes in burnout and satisfaction with work-life integration in physicians during the first 2 years of the COVID-19 pandemic. *Mayo Clin Proc*. 2022;97(12):2248–2258. https://doi.org/10.1016/j.mayocp.2022.09.002

10. Kim A, Novinson D. Most clinicians don't want their kids to work in medicine. Interest is booming anyway. *Doximity*. February 23, 2022. Accessed March 20, 2024. https://opmed.doximity.com/articles/most-clinicians-don-t-want-their-kids-to-work-in-medicine-interest-is-booming-anyway

2 Your New White Coat

In chapter 1, we explored the emotional forces that motivated you to pursue a career in medicine. In particular, we explored how your decision was influenced by a drive to satisfy different emotional needs. In this chapter, we will uncover how the journey to become a physician fundamentally changed you.

Medical school was a period during which you spent countless hours studying the inner workings of the human body. You absorbed a vast amount of information, the majority of which you have forgotten. Unless you are a surgeon, you no longer remember the origin, innervation or blood supply of every muscle. I also doubt there is a single practicing clinician who remembers the steps of the Krebs cycle. Nevertheless, medical school accomplished its mission which was to teach you how to reason through a large quantity of clinical information to develop a differential diagnosis and treatment plan.

This process continued during residency. The only difference was you honed in on the intricate details of your specialty. Considering how much clinical information is covered in any specialty, odds are you have also forgotten a fair share of what you learned at this stage of your training.

While you were intensely focused on gaining the necessary knowledge and skills to practice clinical medicine, another simultaneous process was transpiring during medical training. It was subtle and hidden from plain sight. Yet, it had an equally profound impact on you. You were unknowingly undergoing a radical transformation to fit the mold of a physician. Your way of thinking and behaving subconsciously changed every time you interacted with colleagues and attending physicians.

If you doubt this, consider how much you emotionally changed between the start and end of your medical training. The transformation is remarkable. You have put on a new white coat that creates a chasm between you and those outside medicine. A resident physician described this experience as she was preparing to graduate. She described feeling like she had

DOI: 10.4324/9781003473923-4

nothing in common with people who did not work in medicine. During social gatherings, she did not know how to contribute to conversations because the vast majority of her past and present life experiences revolved around medicine. Even when people would politely ask her about her career, she kept her responses superficial knowing they could not relate to her life journey.

To some degree, this is understandable. People without a clinical background cannot relate to your journey. They have not walked in your footsteps or endured your sacrifices. They do not understand what it is like to study for board exams while working 80 hours per week. They have not been exposed to the amount of illness, injury and death that you have witnessed. Nor have they felt the pressure and responsibility of making clinical decisions that determine a human being's fate.

Though isolating, your transformation during training was necessary. Being a physician entails more than simply knowing how to diagnose and treat different health conditions. You also need to possess certain attributes to practice medicine. For example, you need to be capable of maintaining your composure to intervene effectively in high-stakes situations. You also need to maintain laser focus and pay close attention to details. Even the slightest mistake when writing a prescription or performing a surgical procedure can have lethal consequences.

As a result, medicine favors applicants with certain traits, which it further cultivates during training. Consider the personality trait of conscientiousness, which has been found to be a significant predictor of performance during medical school (1). It benefits patient care if physicians demonstrate a strong desire to do a good job and take their responsibilities seriously. In addition, the subscales of responsibility, tolerance, sociability and self-acceptance from the California Personality Inventory have emerged as predictors of success in medical training (2).

Despite its potential benefits in clinical settings, the process of selecting for and fostering specific traits can inadvertently come with negative consequences, especially when traits are cultivated to the extreme or at the expense of other ones. As described by Aristotle, it is the golden mean, the intermediate zone between the polar ends of excess and deficiency, in which virtuous behavior occurs (3).

For example, empathy, which is the ability to emotionally understand what someone is experiencing, is associated with improved clinical outcomes and patient satisfaction (4, 5, 6). As a result, medical schools favor applicants demonstrating high levels of this virtue or personality traits positively associated with it such as agreeableness and conscientiousness (7).

However, empathy comes with potential pitfalls. Overidentifying with a patient's suffering can interfere with clinical judgment. Focusing too much on someone's plight and being emotionally carried away by it can prevent you from being objective when deciding on the proper course of action. In addition, it has been suggested that empathy is associated with burnout because it draws on one's mental resources (8).

Furthermore, empathy can be associated with lapses in ethical judgment. Connecting intensely with someone's emotional experience can predispose you to overlooking and justifying their transgressions. Evidence shows that empathy is not free from bias. In general, we are less likely to empathize with people from different racial and cultural groups, which can exacerbate the bias plaguing medicine (9).

As an additional example, conscientiousness is not always a beneficial trait, even though medicine selects for it. Being overly conscientious can slow you down and reduce your productivity (10). This can be a major hinderance for a medical student who is on the clock during a standardized exam or a physician swamped with a full caseload on a busy clinic day.

These examples highlight that it is important to know yourself on a deeper level because medicine has changed you. Let's explore seven traits that were reinforced during your medical training. Though useful in clinical settings, they can also predispose you to burnout, and other emotional difficulties, especially when cultivated to their extremes.

1. Selflessness

The cardinal rule of medicine is that the patient always comes first. This is a sound principle because patients are in a vulnerable position when they seek our services. There is a significant knowledge gap and they rely on us to make clinical decisions that are in their best interest. Prioritizing their needs over yours protects them from exploitation and serves as the foundation of the patient-physician relationship.

The problem occurs when selflessness becomes synonymous with self-sacrifice. Medicine praises physicians who go the extra mile for their patients and colleagues. It idealizes the surgeon who was able to endure a long surgical case or the family doctor who saw 30 patients in a day. In such an environment, practicing self-care feels prohibitive. Being surrounded by competitive, achievement-oriented perfectionists who work non-stop only intensifies the guilt associated with basic self-care.

2. Obedience

One of the traits that helped you complete medical school and residency was your ability to figure out and adapt to the expectations of different supervising physicians. Being obedient spared you many troubles during medical training.

Some supervisors wanted you to write the most meticulous notes and would be critical if you left out any information, even if it was not pertinent to the diagnosis and treatment plan. Other supervisors would criticize you for being too wordy and want your notes to get to the point. The ability to adapt to a supervisor's expectations was critical to survive training. Defying their expectations could result in negative reviews and retaliation.

Due to its hierarchical nature, medicine is characterized by power differences which can lead to abuse and boundary violations. A resident described to me how an attending approached her the week before a deadline to submit a presentation for a conference. The resident politely declined because the request was on short notice. She was in the midst of a grueling rotation and struggling to keep up with its demands. She barely had enough time to meet her basic needs, let alone write up a proposal.

When she declined, the attending replied "I'm disappointed in you" and retaliated by being more demanding and critical in future interactions.

The expectation to be an obedient team player only continues as an attending physician. You are expected to accommodate your employer's demands. Any time a hospital goes through financial hardship, the reflex is to ask physicians to be more productive and generate more revenue or suffer a reduction in compensation. Due to years of conditioning, your initial instinct is to be obedient by reflexively acquiescing to their demands even if you are already burned out from working to the max.

3. High-Achieving

Medicine is a field that attracts high-achievers. My academic performance stood out in college as I graduated *Summa Cum Laude*. This changed in medical school where I was surrounded by classmates with more impressive resumes from prestigious colleges.

In such a hypercompetitive environment, you have no choice but to join the hamster wheel of working harder and longer. Falling behind can make you look bad in the eyes of supervising physicians resulting in negative performance reviews. If your classmate is volunteering to work on the weekends or staying up until 2 am to write a case report, then not keeping up with them does not bode well for you.

Being surrounded by high-achievers changes you. It increases your need to achieve because you compare yourself to peers who also have a high need to achieve. The outcome is that you become obsessed with achievement and prioritize it over everything else including your health and relationship with loved ones. Taking a break is a challenge not only due to the time demands of medical training. Emotional forces such as shame and guilt prevent you from jumping off the hamster wheel of achievement.

Your need to achieve is on steroids. You have raised your bar of expectations to the point that being a physician no longer feels like an achievement.

4. Stoicism

The culture of medicine promotes stoicism. To some degree, this is understandable. On a daily basis, we make decisions that impact the quality of one's life. These high-stakes decisions can be quite stressful. The last thing you want is to have your emotions cloud your clinical judgment and harm a patient. As a result, you are proficient in pushing your emotions aside to focus on the task at hand.

Like any other trait, suppression is a double-edged sword. You can bottle or ignore your feelings for only so long before they return with a vengeance and negatively impact you. I have worked with many physicians who were able to keep their emotions in check at work but would blow up at home at the drop of a dime.

There comes a time when you have to identify and process your thoughts and feelings. This is the equivalent of loosening the valve on a tense pipe to release the built-up pressure before it bursts. Unfortunately, medicine has failed to provide you with the time, space and skillset to engage in this meaningful practice. As a result, you do your best to cope by taking a stoic stance and ignoring how you feel.

5. Self-Sufficiency

Medicine has trained you to be self-sufficient. This trait can come in handy when you are on your own and need to rapidly act on a differential diagnosis and treatment plan. You may be responsible for treating an unconscious patient during an emergency or someone who is a poor historian. Being self-sufficient helps you be resourceful and come up with solutions in the face of uncertainty.

When taken to the extreme, self-sufficiency is not compatible with asking for help. One has to relinquish control and rely on someone else for help. This can be difficult when you are used to having the final word in making clinical decisions.

The truth is that medicine is a collaborative profession. It is in the best interest of our patients that we work together. There are times when you need to consult a colleague who may be more skilled in addressing a particular health problem. Not seeking appropriate help can hinder patient care.

Finally, never asking for help due to a need to be in control is a surefire way to have your life spiral out of control due to carrying too many responsibilities. The ability to delegate tasks appropriately is important in establishing work-life balance.

6. Perfectionism

Medicine is unforgiving when mistakes occur. To this day, I vividly remember my chief resident screaming at me when I made a mistake during sign-out. Even though it was my first week as an intern, I can understand his reaction. Errors can have catastrophic outcomes for the patient. In many clinical scenarios, anything less than perfection is simply not an acceptable outcome. As a result, medicine reinforces perfectionism.

The problem is that perfectionism is associated with a host of mental health difficulties such as depression, anxiety, eating disorders and even suicidal ideation (11, 12). It is also a risk factor for physician burnout. A cross-sectional study of physicians in a children's hospital network found that perfectionism contributed to the emotional exhaustion and depersonalization dimensions of burnout (13). This is consistent with broader literature outside medicine showing a link between perfectionism and burnout (14).

Perfectionists have a tendency of setting their bar of expectations at unsustainable levels. They carry immense pressure to meet high standards of performance. Though well-intentioned, such expectations make them prone to emotional difficulties.

7. Grit

You would have not made it through the odyssey of medical training without grit. Medicine attracts individuals with type A personality traits who are highly competitive, driven and goal-oriented. According to a cross-sectional study of practicing physicians, 53% of participants identified as workaholics and 62% as having type A Personality (15). I bet the remaining participants of the study were also type A workaholics but did not know it. It can be hard to engage in accurate self-reflection when you are surrounded by people who also carry your traits.

Having a strong work ethic is essential to survive medical training. During residency, my call shifts lasted 30 hours. I would not have survived those shifts without grit. At the end of one of those shifts, I felt particularly tired which I expressed to a seasoned attending. He proceeded to tell me how easy I had it as he recounted with nostalgia his training which entailed longer and more frequent call shifts. His response was a clear message that any expression of discontent would not be tolerated.

Physicians are well accustomed to working to the point of exhaustion. However, even grit can be hazardous when taken to the extreme. I worked with a physician who showed up to work with a fever, chills and body aches. They must have appeared quite ill because one of their colleagues escorted them to the Emergency Department for further care.

In medicine, grit has become synonymous with a complete neglect of one's needs and overall health. It is ironic that we preach to our patients the importance of self-care and healthy habits, but don't come even close to practicing this in our personal and professional lives.

The Outcome

Medicine may be well-intended in selecting for selfless, hard-working, achievement-oriented, lifelong learners who will move heaven and earth to address a patient's health concern. Cultivating these traits promotes patient care. However, the manner in which medicine reinforces these traits needs to change because it makes medical students and physicians vulnerable to burnout and mental health difficulties.

Evidence shows that burnout becomes prevalent early in one's medical training. A review found that 45%–56% of medical students had symptoms consistent with burnout. Its prevalence increased as students advanced through their training (16). According to a pooled analysis of data from 1,428 fourth year medical students, 49% of respondents had burnout, 38% endorsed depressive symptoms and 34% low mental quality of life (17). This indicates that incoming residents are likely to suffer from substantial burnout and emotional difficulties even before the start of their intern year.

Residency training only exacerbates the problem. According to a systematic review and meta-analysis, the prevalence of depressive symptoms among resident physicians was 28.8% (18). A national survey found that 60% of resident and fellow physicians suffer from burnout (19).

Attributing these trends to the individual entering medicine is a gross misunderstanding of what is transpiring. Matriculating medical students begin training with similar or even better mental health profiles compared to age-matched college graduates pursuing different careers (20). Their mental health deteriorates early in medical school with higher levels of depression and burnout compared to peers outside medicine (19). This indicates there is something inherently problematic about the culture of medicine, its training regimen and work conditions that cause this group of bright, motivated and resilient individuals to experience a deterioration of their mental health.

Your new white coat might help you care for patients. However, it also makes you vulnerable to exploitation even as an attending physician. Your current job operates under the same unwritten rules that you followed during training. You are an obedient employee who reluctantly acquiesces to increasing demands from hospital administrators even if you are already working at maximum capacity. You do not speak up for fear of retribution. Despite experiencing difficulties, you do not ask for help for fear of appearing weak. You rely on stoicism to cope with your current set of circumstances and bottle up for feelings. Your reflex is to work harder and longer by digging deep into your mental reserves in search of more strength and perseverance. Only now you are older with years of wear and tear and lack the stamina of your youthful years.

What worked in the past is not serving you today. Being obedient might have helped you survive training. However, blind obedience only makes you vulnerable to exploitation by institutions adopting big business practices. You have been conditioned to feel and act like a trainee who needs to report to an authority figure. Perpetuating this cycle is not in your best interest. As an attending physician, you carry more autonomy and authority than you realize. You have options because you are in demand. You have clinical expertise and experience that is hard to find.

It is time to embrace who you are and shed the white coat you were prescribed. It no longer serves you. Discarding your white coat might sound intimidating because you have worn it for so long. However, it is the only way to stop your current spiral of burnout and prioritize your mental health.

References

1. Doherty EM, Nugent E. Personality factors and medical training: a review of the literature. *Med Educ*. 2011;45(2):132–140. doi:10.1111/j.1365-2923.2010.03760.x
2. Ferguson E, James D, Madeley L. Factors associated with success in medical school: systematic review of the literature. *BMJ*. 2002;324(7343):952–957. doi:10.1136/bmj.324.7343.952
3. Kraut, R. Stanford encyclopedia of philosophy: Aristotle's ethics. 2001. Accessed March 24, 2024. https://plato.stanford.edu/entries/aristotle-ethics/#VirtDefiC ontInco
4. Del Canale S, Louis DZ, Maio V, et al. The relationship between physician empathy and disease complications: an empirical study of primary care physicians and their diabetic patients in Parma, Italy. *Acad Med*. 2012;87(9):1243–1249. doi:10.1097/ACM.0b013e3182628fbf
5. Hojat M, Louis DZ, Markham FW, Wender R, Rabinowitz C, Gonnella JS. Physicians' empathy and clinical outcomes for diabetic patients. *Acad Med*. 2011;86(3):359–364. doi:10.1097/ACM.0b013e3182086fe1
6. Kirby R, Knowles HC, Patel A, et al. The influence of patient perception of physician empathy on patient satisfaction among attending physicians working with residents in an emergent care setting. *Health Sci Rep*. 2021 Aug 17;4(3):e337. doi:10.1002/hsr2.337

7. Melchers MC, Li M, Haas BW, Reuter M, Bischoff L, Montag C. Similar personality patterns are associated with empathy in four different countries. *Front Psychol*. 2016 Mar 8;7:290. doi:10.3389/fpsyg.2016.00290

8. Wilkinson H, Whittington R, Perry L, Eames C. Examining the relationship between burnout and empathy in healthcare professionals: a systematic review. *Burn Res*. 2017;6:18–29. doi:10.1016/j.burn.2017.06.003

9. Cikara M, Bruneau E, Van Bavel JJ, Saxe R. Their pain gives us pleasure: how intergroup dynamics shape empathic failures and counter-empathic responses. *J Exp Soc Psychol*. 2014;55:110–125. doi:10.1016/j.jesp.2014.06.007

10. Tett, R. Is conscientiousness always positively related to job performance. *TIP*. 1998;36(1). https://www.researchgate.net/publication/288166009_Is_conscientiousness_always_positively_related_to_job_performance

11. Egan SJ, Wade TD, Shafran R. Perfectionism as a transdiagnostic process: a clinical review. *Clinical Psychology Review*. 2011;31(2):203–212. https://doi.org/10.1016/j.cpr.2010.04.009

12. Flett GL, Hewitt PL, Heisel MJ. The destructiveness of perfectionism revisited: implications for the assessment of suicide risk and the prevention of suicide. *Review of General Psychology*. 2014 Sept;18(3):156–172. doi:10.1037/gpr0000011

13. Martin SR, Fortier MA, Heyming TW, et al. Perfectionism as a predictor of physician burnout. *BMC Health Serv Res*. 2022 Nov 28;22:1425. doi:10.1186/s12913-022-08785-7

14. Hill AP, Curran T. Multidimensional perfectionism and burnout: a meta-analysis. *Personality and Social Psychology Review*. 2016;20(3):269–288. https://doi.org/10.1177/1088868315596286

15. Lemaire JB, Wallace JE. How physicians identify with predetermined personalities and links to perceived performance and wellness outcomes: a cross-sectional study. *BMC Health Serv Res*. 2014;14:616. https://doi.org/10.1186/s12913-014-0616-z

16. Dyrbye L, Shanafelt T. A narrative review on burnout experienced by medical students and residents. *Med Educ*. 2016;50(1):132–149. doi:10.1111/medu.12927

17. Dyrbye LN, Moutier C, Durning SJ, et al. The problems program directors inherit: medical student distress at the time of graduation. *Med Teach*. 2011;33(9):756–758. doi:10.3109/0142159X.2011.577468

18. Mata DA, Ramos MA, Bansal N, et al. Prevalence of depression and depressive symptoms among resident physicians: a systematic review and meta-analysis. *JAMA*. 2015;314(22):2373–2383. https://doi.org/10.1001/jama.2015.15845

19. Dyrbye LN, West CP, Satele D, et al. Burnout among U.S. medical students, residents, and early career physicians relative to the general U.S. population. *Acad Med*. 2014;89(3):443–451. doi:10.1097/ACM.0000000000000134

20. Brazeau CM, Shanafelt T, Durning SJ, et al. Distress among matriculating medical students relative to the general population. *Acad Med*. 2014;89(11):1520–1525. doi:10.1097/ACM.0000000000000482

3 You Have Been Traumatized

Imagine you had a magic wand and could practice medicine in an ideal setting. You did not have to deal with insurance companies declining coverage for prescribed treatments. There were no hospital administrators breathing down your neck for failing to meet productivity or patient satisfaction benchmarks. You had generous time to work on meaningful research and quality improvement projects that could positively impact patient care. The electronic medical record was a welcome asset that helped you document and coordinate patient care rather than a distraction during clinical encounters. You practiced medicine without the fear of litigation looming over you like a gray cloud. You could leave work at a reasonable time to be with loved ones rather than spend your evenings documenting clinical encounters.

Let's assume you were a unicorn and practiced medicine in an ideal setting. My question is would you still be at risk of burnout in this hypothetical scenario?

The answer is yes.

Practicing medicine is inherently challenging, even in ideal settings. What makes it hard is not only the volume but also the nature of the work. We have a front row seat to human suffering and are exposed to traumatic events at a high frequency. These include treating patients with critical injuries or illnesses, helping victims of physical, emotional and sexual abuse, being the victims of workplace violence, witnessing the death of patients and coping with the fear of exposure to potentially lethal viruses such as during the COVID pandemic. In a study of 1,134 interns, 56.4% reported exposure to traumatic events during their internship. The rate of exposure ranged from 43.1% to 72.4% depending on the specialty (1).

Please note this study highlights the trauma physicians were exposed to during a single year of practicing medicine. Imagine the amount of trauma that a physician is exposed to throughout their entire career.

DOI: 10.4324/9781003473923-5

Working closely with physicians has taught me that exposure to traumatic events in medicine comes at a great emotional toll. As an example, I worked with a resident who was experiencing sleep disturbances during her Emergency Medicine rotation. On the surface, it would be easy to attribute her complaint to the fluctuating work schedule of the rotation. Switching between working day and night shifts can disrupt sleep.

However, it is important to test underlying assumptions rather than jump to premature conclusions. I asked the resident whether her sleep was interrupted by distressing dreams which was the case. She described a disturbing dream that would wake her up multiple times per week. It involved the image of an adolescent whose skin and tissue had been torn off their scalp revealing their underlying skull. Upon further inquiry, the resident reported that she had recently treated an unconscious adolescent with a devastating degloving injury from a motor vehicle accident. She recalled feeling both horrified and helpless at the sight of the gruesome injury. Despite the distressing feelings, she was able to maintain her composure during the case and for the remainder of her shift. However, the traumatic event had left its mark. A few days after this case, she noticed a spike in anxiety when driving due to the fear of being seriously injured in a motor vehicle accident.

On the surface, this resident was performing well. Nobody in her residency program knew anything was wrong. She was providing quality patient care and not exhibiting any evidence of a mental health disturbance. Behind her veil of stoicism, I could see cracks in her psychological armor. It was only a matter of time before further exposure to traumatic events would disrupt her ability to function at work and home.

By promoting a culture of stoicism, medicine has failed to appreciate how traumatic experiences impact healthcare providers. Medicine holds a narrow view on the impact of trauma. The ability to take appropriate and timely action during a high-stakes event is interpreted as evidence that the physician is unscathed and can continue with their responsibilities as usual. However, one's performance at work is not necessarily an accurate metric of one's well-being. Physicians are adept at concealing their thoughts and feelings while completing a task at hand. The effects from being exposed to trauma are often not apparent until a later time when they can no longer keep their guard up. This usually happens in settings outside medicine. Hence, colleagues may be surprised to hear that a physician is struggling when they may appear to function well at work.

What is Trauma?

Medicine has traditionally held a narrow view of what constitutes trauma. It has been synonymous with a threat to one's physical well-being such as a cardiovascular event, serious injuries following a physical assault or motor vehicle accident, or death. However, the American Psychological Association defines trauma as "any disturbing experience that results in significant fear, helplessness, dissociation, confusion, or other disruptive feelings intense enough to have a long-lasting negative effect on a person's attitudes, behavior, and other aspects of functioning." It also notes that traumatic events "often challenge the individual's view of the world as a just, safe and predictable place" (2).

Think about how often this happens in medicine. Depending on your specialty, you may be exposed to "disturbing experiences" that result in "disruptive feelings intense enough to have a long-lasting negative impact" on a daily basis. Regardless of your specialty, you are exposed, either directly or indirectly, to traumatic stress which is strongly associated with occupational burnout (3). Such exposure also makes you vulnerable to different mental health conditions such as posttraumatic stress disorder (PTSD), which is characterized by a constellation of symptoms including intrusive nightmares and flashbacks, avoidance of trauma-related reminders, negative thoughts and feelings, difficulty with sleep and concentration, a negative perception of oneself and the world, being prone to irritability, an exaggerated startle response and hypervigilance. The same study of 1,134 interns found that 19.0% of those who experienced trauma screened positive for PTSD and the 12-month PTSD rates of training physicians were three times greater than the general population (1). A different study of practicing Emergency Medicine physicians showed the prevalence of self-assessed PTSD was 15.8%, which is more than four times the point prevalence of PTSD in U.S. adults (4).

Trauma from Clinical Encounters

Another misconception in medicine is that you are only impacted by traumatic events that you directly encounter. In other words, trauma only has an effect if you are physically affected or witness it with your own eyes. As illustrated by the case of the resident who treated a patient with a degloving injury, direct exposure to trauma can have a profound emotional impact on even the most resilient physician.

However, even indirect exposure, such as when patients share details of personal traumatic experiences, can negatively impact you. Vicarious traumatization refers to negative changes in a clinician's view of themselves, others, and the world stemming from repeated empathic engagement with patients' trauma-related thoughts, memories and emotions (5). Repeatedly listening with empathy to stories of human suffering can diminish feelings of safety by magnifying the dangers of the surrounding environment. It is an emotionally challenging experience when patients project their fears onto you. You can be exposed to their thoughts and feelings for only so long before you start to emotionally wear out or detach during the patient encounter, which are classic symptoms of burnout.

As an example, I worked with a physician who presented following the sudden passing of a family member. They went to check on them after they did not come down for dinner. When repeated calls to open their bedroom door went unanswered, they broke through the door only to find them deceased. The physician described in horrifying detail their desperate attempt to revive them by performing CPR.

Even though I was not the victim of this tragedy and did not directly witness it, it had an emotional impact on me. I remember feeling my throat tighten while listening to gory details of the case. Despite sitting in a comfortable chair, I could feel my heart pounding through my chest. Sweat was dripping down my dress shirt as if I had run a dead sprint. I felt overwhelmed by the abrupt nature and magnitude of the tragedy.

A sense of desperation overcame me as I wanted to help the human being who was crying inconsolably in front of me. There was nothing I could do to bring back their loved one or make their pain go away. No words could capture the magnitude of their suffering. All I could do in that moment was give them the necessary space and time to freely express their thoughts and feelings about their loss. Remembering that empathy can be healing served as my compass during the session. In the words of a mentor, *"Listening with empathy is doing. Say less and listen more."*

I tried to emotionally understand what my patient was going through by imagining myself in their shoes. I thought about how terrified and devastated I would have felt if I ever found a loved one in a lifeless state. I imagined the desperation of performing CPR to revive them. What I was feeling during the session was a mere microcosm of how deeply they were suffering. I am fortunate that my feelings during such encounters stem from disturbing fragments of my imagination and emotional projections from patients. I can escape them by grounding myself back to reality. Unfortunately, many of our patients are not afforded the same opportunity and remain trapped in the nightmare of their realities.

Such encounters are common in medicine. You have had many patients open up to share details of their traumatic experiences. They might have spoken to you about physical, emotional or sexual abuse they have encountered or feelings stemming from the abrupt loss of a loved one. Such encounters leave a scar even if you have not been the direct victim of the abuse or loss. They are painful reminders of the dangers and fragility that define the human condition.

Not meeting criteria for PTSD or any other mental health condition does not negate the gravity and impact of exposure to trauma. I have worked with plenty of physicians who used our time in therapy to share their thoughts and feelings about what they witnessed at work. Witnessing the death of an infant, trying to save a critically ill patient bleeding from different orifices, listening to the piecing screech of a burn victim writhing in agony or consoling an abused child can be too much to bear alone.

A negative clinical outcome can intensify the emotional impact of a traumatic encounter. Due to our altruistic nature as physicians, we expect to help and heal every patient we serve. As a result, we often blame ourselves for negative outcomes even if we are not at fault. A systematic review of over 11,000 healthcare providers involved in adverse events found that the majority experienced a wide range of psychological symptoms such as troubling memories, anxiety, anger towards themselves, fear of future errors, embarrassment, distress, and guilt (6).

Trauma from Physician Encounters

Unfortunately, emotionally difficult clinical cases are not the only source of trauma in medicine. What is most troubling is that colleagues and faculty members can be a source of trauma. Sexual harassment is prevalent in medicine due to its hierarchical structure which creates discrepancies in power, pay and leadership opportunities. A study of over 3,300 full-time faculty from 24 U.S. medical schools found that about half of female faculty had experienced some form of sexual harassment. It also found that female faculty were at least 2.5 times more likely to experience gender-based discrimination compared to their male counterparts (7). Unfortunately, sexual harassment is a pervasive problem beginning in the earliest stages of training when power differences are most notable. A multisite study of medical students found that 36.6% of them reported experiencing sexual harassment behavior by a faculty/staff member. The study also found that those who experienced sexual harassment were more likely to endorse symptoms of PTSD and depression (8).

It is ironic that we enter medicine with the purest intention to heal those suffering from health problems. Yet, medicine compromises the health and safety of its own by subjecting them to traumatic experiences such as sexual harassment, bias and discrimination. Acts of microaggression are also embedded within the fabric of medicine and glorified as rites of passage. An example includes residents being pimped during rounds on the clinical details of a case and humiliated for not knowing an answer.

Adverse Childhood Experiences

We do not enter medicine as a blank slate. Some of our past life experiences are quite painful and impact how we perceive and respond to traumatic events we encounter in medicine.

Exposure to trauma often begins in childhood. The Adverse Childhood Experiences (ACE) study, which included responses from over 9,500 adults who had completed a standardized medical evaluation at a large health maintenance organization (HMO), found that more than half of respondents experienced at least one type of ACE. It also found a strong graded positive association between the number of childhood exposures to adverse events and the prevalence of different leading causes of death in adulthood including smoking, obesity, physical inactivity, depressed mood, suicide attempts, alcoholism and illicit drug use (9). A more recent study found that nearly 16% of adults had experienced four or more types of ACE (10).

As physicians, we are not exempt from this reality. We enter the profession with our own set of challenging, and often painful, past life experiences. A study of physicians found that 49% of them had experienced at least one ACE, while 9% four or more ACEs. The study also found that physicians who reported higher burnout were more likely to have higher underlying ACE scores (11). This association is understandable when you consider that common symptoms of burnout—including mental exhaustion, helplessness and detachment—can also be manifestations of traumatic stress (12).

Our past influences our perception of current stressors and ability to respond to them. We often witness events that hit too close to home. Pointing out this influence is not intended to minimize the impact of systemic factors, which are the primary drivers of physician burnout. Nor is it intended to minimize how emotionally difficult it is to work in the front lines of human suffering or excuse physicians who misuse their positions of authority to prey on more vulnerable colleagues.

On the contrary, acknowledging the widespread and profound impact of trauma is intended to highlight less-known factors that contribute to the burnout epidemic and emphasize the importance of adopting a more comprehensive approach that is informed by trauma principles. The narrative regarding burnout needs to evolve. Though less known, exposure to trauma has a negative impact on physicians. In addition to eradicating the systemic factors plaguing medicine, there needs to be an emphasis on implementing principles and policies that make medicine a less traumatic and more humane working environment.

Trauma-Informed Care

Trauma-informed care (TIC) refers to an organizational framework that seeks to promote safety within medicine, support those exposed to trauma and prevent future traumatization by recognizing the different manifestations of trauma and their impact on physicians, patients and the entire healthcare system. TIC promotes structural and cultural change within an organization by addressing evidence-based drivers of physician burnout and promoting evidence-based protective factors such as the cultivation of community and collaboration. Organizational interventions guided by principles of TIC have been shown to reduce burnout and improve employee effectiveness (13).

The need for widespread organizational changes that address the prevalence and impact of trauma in healthcare further reinforces the concept that suffering from burnout is not your fault. Stop blaming yourself for your struggles or thinking that suffering is a sign of weakness.

You are plenty resilient. Any individual can endure only so many traumatic encounters before they start to break down. Each traumatic encounter is the equivalent of tearing a thread off a rope that is holding a heavy weight. The effect from a single tear may not be noticeable. However, the rope, regardless of how resilient it is, can endure only so many tears before it completely rips apart and drops the weight. No physician is exempt from this reality.

Even though you are not to blame for your suffering, you are responsible for navigating the difficult hand you have been dealt. Do not be a bystander waiting for the system to implement trauma-informed policies that humanize the culture of medicine. When traumatic stress triggers feelings of helplessness, the reflex is to shut down and dissociate (14). Unfortunately, this response does not solve any of your problems. It only diminishes your ability to navigate current and future stressors, which is a problem in itself.

Taking action in the face of adversity is the most effective path forward. This starts with speaking up and advocating for yourself. Do not settle for an employer who does not prioritize physician well-being and patient care. Job security is not worth betraying the values you stand for. Remember you are a physician and in high demand. Explore your options. You will find positions better aligned with your vision of how medicine should be practiced.

Also, do not stay silent when a colleague mistreats you. Silence only perpetuates the mistreatment by letting perpetrators off the hook. Speak up by informing the proper channels at your institution. Perpetrators need to face consequences for their actions. If you are in a position of authority, you have a moral duty to advocate for those with less leverage.

Exposure to trauma, either directly or indirectly, is inevitable when practicing clinical medicine. Organizations have a responsibility to implement policies and practices that protect physicians from its effects. In the meantime, recognize how such exposure impacts your personal life and take the proper course of action to mitigate its effect. Resist the urge to stay silent or ignore the problem. This approach will not work. Your best bet is to speak up against perpetrators, mobilize your support system and even seek professional help to navigate exposure to traumatic events when practicing clinical medicine.

References

1. Vance MC, Mash HBH, Ursano RJ, et al. Exposure to workplace trauma and posttraumatic stress disorder among intern physicians. *JAMA Netw Open*. 2021;4(6):e2112837. doi:10.1001/jamanetworkopen.2021.12837
2. APA Dictionary of Psychology. *American Psychological Association*. April 2018. Accessed April 7, 2024. https://dictionary.apa.org/trauma
3. Cieslak R, Shoji K, Douglas A, Melville E, Luszczynska A, Benight CC. A meta-analysis of the relationship between job burnout and secondary traumatic stress among workers with indirect exposure to trauma. *Psychol Serv*. 2014 Feb;11(1):75–86. doi:10.1037/a0033798. Epub 2013 Aug 12. PMID:23937082
4. DeLucia JA, Bitter C, Fitzgerald J, Greenberg M, Dalwari P, Buchanan P. Prevalence of post-traumatic stress disorder in emergency physicians in the United States. *West J Emerg Med*. 2019 Aug 28;20(5):740–746. doi:10.5811/westjem.2019.7.42671. PMID:31539331; PMCID:PMC6754196
5. Quitangton, G. Vicarious trauma in clinicians: fostering resilience and preventing burnout. *Psychiatric Times*. 2019 July 26;36(7). Accessed April 6, 2024. https://www.psychiatrictimes.com/view/vicarious-trauma-clinicians-fostering-resilience-and-preventing-burnout
6. Busch IM, Moretti F, Purgato M, Barbui C, Wu AW, Rimondini M. Psychological and psychosomatic symptoms of second victims of adverse events: a systematic review and meta-analysis [published correction appears in *J Patient Saf*. 2020 Sept;16(3):e211]. *J Patient Saf*. 2020;16(2):e61–e74. doi:10.1097/PTS.0000000000000589
7. Carr PL, Ash AS, Friedman RH, et al. Faculty perceptions of gender discrimination and sexual harassment in academic medicine. *Ann Intern Med*. 2000;132(11):889–896. doi:10.7326/0003-4819-132-11-200006060-00007
8. McClain T, Kammer-Kerwick M, Wood L, Temple JR, Busch-Armendariz N. Sexual harassment among medical students: prevalence, prediction, and correlated outcomes. *Workplace Health & Safety*. 2021;69(6):257–267. doi:10.1177/2165079920969402
9. Felitti VJ, Anda RF, Nordenberg D, et al. Relationship of childhood abuse and household dysfunction to many of the leading causes of death in adults. The Adverse Childhood Experiences (ACE) Study. *Am J Prev Med*. 1998;14(4):245–258. doi:10.1016/s0749-3797(98)00017-8
10. Merrick MT, Ford DC, Ports KA, et al. Vital signs: estimated proportion of adult health problems attributable to adverse childhood experiences and implications for prevention – 25 states, 2015–2017. *MMWR Morb Mortal Wkly Rep*. 2019 Nov 8;68(44):999–1005. doi:10.15585/mmwr.mm6844e1
11. Yellowlees P, Coate L, Misquitta R, Wetzel AE, Parish MB. The association between adverse childhood experiences and burnout in a regional sample of physicians. *Acad Psychiatry*. 2021 Apr;45(2):159–163. doi:10.1007/s40596-020-01381-z. Epub 2021 Jan 6. PMID:33409937

12. Elisseou S. Trauma-informed care: a missing link in addressing burnout. *J Healthc Leadersh*. 2023;15:169–173. doi:10.2147/JHL.S389271
13. Hales TW, Nochajski TH. A structural regression analysis of trauma-informed climate factors, organizational commitment, and burnout among behavioral healthcare providers in a large public hospital. *J Community Psychol*. 2020;48(3):777–792. doi:10.1002/jcop.22292
14. Schalinski I, Moran J, Schauer M, Elbert T. Rapid emotional processing in relation to trauma-related symptoms as revealed by magnetic source imaging. *BMC Psychiatry*. 2014;14:193. doi:10.1186/1471-244X-14-193

Part 2

Know the System

4 Bias in Medicine

You entered medicine with pure intentions. Your desire to help others by alleviating their suffering played a major role in your decision to become a physician. However, a moral conundrum became apparent early in your training. Bias and discrimination are prevalent among physicians. Even though they are supposed to be pillars of compassion and empathy, physicians contribute to each other's suffering, both knowingly and unknowingly, through their personal belief systems and actions.

During your training, you devoted countless hours studying the intricate details of how the body functions down to the cellular level. You developed the necessary clinical skills to serve your patients. Yet, medicine has a fundamental flaw in its training. It has failed to teach physicians how to have compassion for each other.

Medical education promotes a zero-sum game in which achievement-oriented perfectionists fiercely compete against each other to reach their professional goals. This occurs throughout the entire span of medical training. Competing against your peers is understandable as class ranking, performance on standardized exams and research output determine the trajectory of your medical career and, ultimately, your life.

However, the competitive mindset also comes at a cost. It teaches physicians to compete rather than collaborate with one another. Prioritizing class ranks and percentile scores on standardized exams as the primary drivers of professional success reinforces the idea that you need to be better than peers who are pursuing similar goals. This win-lose mindset creates a vertical hierarchy in which some physicians view themselves as more valuable or superior to others. Unfortunately, this mindset carries beyond medical training and can explain why some physicians engage in behaviors which undermine and even take advantage of their colleagues.

An example of this pattern is turfing, a term used to describe when the transfer of a patient between physicians occurs in an ethically and

DOI: 10.4324/9781003473923-7

clinically problematic manner. What makes turfing problematic is that the primary objective of the transfer is not necessarily to improve patient care. Rather, the physician is transferring the patient to defer the responsibility of caring for them because the perceived trouble outweighs the benefit. Physicians receiving such transfers can feel resentful about the increased workload from the inappropriate transfer. In addition, turfed patients may have more unfavorable care experiences compared to patients who have been appropriately assigned to a medical service (1).

Another problematic outcome of this competitive mindset is that it fails to cultivate an environment in which physicians engage in self-reflection to uncover preexisting biases that may stem from one's familial upbringing, cultural background and socioeconomic status. Medical students and resident physicians barely have enough time to scarf down a sandwich during their work shifts, let alone engage in reflective introspection to explore personal beliefs and understand how they influence their interactions with peers or patients. The outcome of this reality is that we have become so focused on achieving individual professional goals that we fail to appreciate the humanity in each other. This translates into a lack compassion among physicians which creates fertile ground for bias and discrimination to grow and plague the culture of medicine.

Physicians are often the victims of bias and discriminatory behavior from a variety of sources. A cross-sectional study of 6,512 U.S. physicians found that mistreatment and discrimination by patients, families and visitors were common, especially for female physicians and members of racial and ethnic minorities. In particular, 29.4% of participants reported being subjected to racially or ethnically offensive remarks, 28.7% to offensive sexist remarks and 20.5% to unwanted sexual advances at least once in the previous year. In addition, more than one in five physicians (21.6%) reported refusal of care by a patient or their family at least once in the previous year due to the physician's attributes. Exposure to mistreatment and discriminatory behavior was a risk factor for physician burnout (2).

There is no room for prejudice in medicine. It is important that patient and visitor conduct is monitored to protect physicians from discriminatory behaviors. Hospitals should develop protocols for handling such situations. However, it is even more important that, as physicians, we pay close attention to how we treat each other. The majority of physicians experience discrimination from their own colleagues. Shedding light on this problem and taking steps to eradicate it is essential to reduce physician burnout.

Here are some examples of bias and discrimination against different groups of physicians.

Bias against Women

Burnout is more prevalent in female physicians compared to male physicians. According to a survey of over 9,100 U.S. physicians, 63% of female physicians reported burnout compared to 48% of male physicians (3). This finding should not be surprising when you consider the bias against female physicians, which manifests in a number of ways.

First of all, female physicians are placed in the unfair position of carrying the majority of home responsibilities. According to a survey of 1,049 academic physicians, married or partnered women with children spend 8.5 hours more per week on domestic activities compared to married or partnered men. In addition, women are more likely to take time off work during disruptions of usual childcare arrangements (4). Such disruptions can interfere with career advancement because they negatively impact clinical productivity and research output.

The bias against women is further evidenced by the persistent salary gap between women and men. A study of over 10,200 faculty physicians in the U.S. from 24 different medical schools found that women earn annually nearly $20,000 less than men even after adjusting for a number of factors that could account for such a discrepancy such as faculty rank, age, years since residency, specialty, NIH funding, clinical trial participation and publication (5). Being offered lower starting salaries puts women in the unfavorable negotiating position of climbing a larger mountain to advocate for benefits that are offered without reservation to their male counterparts.

Furthermore, women are less likely to hold positions of leadership. According to a cross-sectional study of over 91,000 faculty physicians, women are less likely than men to be full professors, even after accounting for different measures of clinical experience and research productivity. This discrepancy is seen in nearly all medical specialties (6). The shortage of women in leadership roles serves as a barrier to career advancement.

The gender disparity in compensation and career advancement is not based on objective metrics. Studies show that female physicians spend more time with their patients during encounters and earn higher patient satisfaction scores (7). A population-based retrospective cohort study of over 1 million patients found that patients treated by female surgeons had lower rates of adverse postoperative outcomes compared to those treated by male surgeons (8).

There is a glimmer of hope for the future. In 2022, women made up 53.8% of all medical students. As women continue to make up a larger portion of the physician workforce, greater emphasis will be placed in addressing the gender bias which should have been eradicated a long time ago (9).

Bias against International Medical Graduates

International medical graduates (IMGs) account for about 25% of practicing physicians in the U.S. Their diverse clinical and cultural backgrounds enrich the U.S. healthcare system. By receiving their training outside the U.S., IMGs reduce the impact of the physician shortage in a cost-effective manner.

Unfortunately, they face discrimination because some residency programs view them as less competent. As a result, they try to limit the number of IMGs on their roster by either refusing to admit any non-U.S. applicants or establishing strict quota systems that limit the number they accept regardless of qualifications (10).

Viewing IMGs as inferior to U.S. graduates is not based on any objective data. Such perceptions stem from bias. IMGs are required to pass the same medical knowledge standardized exams as U.S. medical school graduates and travel to the U.S. to pass a clinical skills assessment. They are also required to pass a standardized language exam to prove language proficiency.

IMGs certainly face unique challenges when they transition to residency compared to U.S. medical school graduates. They have to adjust to a new culture and learn how to navigate laws, values and treatment modalities that differ from the healthcare system in which they obtained their medical training. Nevertheless, such differences do not make IMGs less competent. They are a vital part of the physician workforce and the discrimination they encounter when applying to residency programs needs to end.

Bias against Racial and Ethnic Minorities

The U.S. has a long and dark history of discrimination against racial and ethnic minorities. Unfortunately, medicine is not exempt from this disturbing history.

The Tuskegee Syphilis study is one of the most egregious examples of medical exploitation against racial minorities. Between 1932 and 1972, hundreds of poor, African American men, the majority of whom had syphilis, were followed to understand the natural course of the disease. Many died as they were not informed of their diagnosis or offered treatment for their condition.

This study is a stark reminder that racism has a devastating effect on clinical judgment and health outcomes. It should also help us empathize with members of racial and ethnic minorities who are hesitant to interact with the healthcare system and seek the care they need. Estimates indicate significantly lower utilization of both outpatient and inpatient medical services by older black men in the years following the study's disclosure (11).

To this day, clinician racial bias negatively influences clinical judgment and predisposes minority groups to inequitable health outcomes. Children from minority groups have longer wait times in the ER (12). Minority adults are less likely to receive catheterization for identical expressions of chest pain (13). Racial and ethnic disparities also exist in pain perception, assessment and treatment across different settings (14).

Physicians from racial and ethnic minorities are not exempt from the discrimination plaguing medicine. A systematic review found they are more likely to experience overt and subtle workplace discrimination from leadership, colleagues and patients. Such discrimination is associated with negative career outcomes, an unwelcoming work environment and feeling isolated (15).

Improving the racial and ethnic diversity of the physician workforce is an essential step to promote health equity. A cross-sectional analysis of over 117,000 Press Ganey surveys found that patients were more satisfied when they experienced racial/ethnic concordance with their physicians (16). As the U.S. population becomes more diverse, it is important that the physician workforce follows a similar evolution with a greater emphasis on patient-centered, culturally-competent care.

There is hope for the future as a 2022 report from the Association of American Medical Colleges showed that the number of applicants and matriculants from underrepresented groups in medicine increased compared to 2020–21. The number of Black or African American applicants increased by 14%, the number of Hispanic applicants by 7.3% and the number of Asian applicants by 13.3%. These trends are an essential step in cultivating a U.S. physician workforce that is more representative of the population and adept in meeting its healthcare needs (9).

Bias Based on Specialty

Physicians also experience discrimination based on their specialty, which is evidenced by the salary difference between primary care physicians and specialists. According to a 2022 survey of more than 10,000 U.S. physicians, specialists earn over $100,000 more annually compared to primary care physicians (17). Despite their critical role as gatekeepers of the healthcare system and drivers of preventative medicine, primary care physicians are grossly underpaid compared to specialists.

However, even specialists discriminate against one another. At one of our therapy sessions, a resident physician shared feeling hurt and ashamed after a resident from a different specialty inquired about future professional goals in the following manner: "Do you still plan on doing butt scopes for a living?"

This comment highlights how physicians can treat each other in a condescending manner. When you have spent your training competing against colleagues, it can be difficult to abandon this mindset and adopt a more collaborative approach in which you appreciate their clinical contributions.

A similar type of bias affects residents who are required to complete a preliminary year of training in internal medicine or general surgery before transitioning to a different residency program to train in their specialty of choice. As an example, I worked with a resident who was wrapping up their preliminary year and looking forward to continuing their training in a different part of the county.

Here is what they said about their experience:

They take more liberties with me because I am leaving at the end of the academic year. I take more call compared to residents who are staying for the entire duration of their training. Chief residents call me to fill last minute gaps on the call schedule. I do my best to stay quiet because I don't want to delay my graduation and start with my new residency program.

Bias Based on Hierarchy

Bias also transpires among physicians of the same specialty based on hierarchy. As resident physicians advance through their training, they obtain leverage over those with fewer years of experience. The way they treat junior residents is often influenced by how they were previously treated by more senior residents.

An intern resident who was on night shifts described a challenging clinical case involving an adolescent with chronic anemia. They presented with an alarmingly low hemoglobin, but were asymptomatic and resting quietly in bed. Never having encountered such a case, the intern consulted with the covering attending physician on call for guidance and followed their recommendations on how to proceed with the case.

When the intern presented the case the following morning during sign-out, senior residents of the medical team were upset and disagreed with how the case was handled. They expressed their disapproval by questioning the intern's competence in a condescending tone. They never gave the intern an opportunity to explain their rationale which was based on recommendations from the attending on-call.

When I asked the intern how they wanted to handle the situation, they were reluctant to bring anything up for fear of retribution from the senior residents. They were concerned that speaking up could compromise opportunities for career advancement.

Outcome

In summary, bias and discrimination are quite prevalent in medicine. The examples in this chapter are only a brief overview of the subject matter. Yet, they highlight a painful truth. The majority of physicians experience some form of discrimination during their training or professional career, often from their own colleagues.

Healthcare organizations must develop policies and practices that promote the diversity of the physician workforce to match the growing diversity of the U.S. population. Such diversity also needs to include a greater emphasis in promoting women and members of racial and ethnic minorities in leadership positions. In addition, policies need to protect physicians from discrimination, regardless of the source. There need to be clear repercussions for physicians who discriminate against colleagues through educational interventions or even penalties depending on the behavior.

At the same time, it is equally important that, as physicians, we treat each other with respect and compassion. Changing the culture of medicine cannot be the sole responsibility of the system. Each one of us has a moral responsibility to speak up when we observe incidents of mistreatment and discriminatory behavior against women and members of racial and ethnic minorities. It is essential that every physician plays an active role in eradicating the discrimination against different groups of physicians.

Finally, please take a moment to explore and address any underlying bias you may carry. It is hurting your colleagues and interfering with the quality of care you provide patients. Improving the healthcare system requires each one of us to look within ourselves to identify areas for improvement. This practice is essential for enhancing our interactions with patients and each other.

References

1. Caldicott CV, Dunn KA, Frankel RM. Can patients tell when they are unwanted? "Turfing" in residency training. *Patient Educ Couns*. 2005;56(1):104–111. doi:10.1016/j.pec.2003.12.014
2. Dyrbye LN, West CP, Sinsky CA, et al. Physicians' experiences with mistreatment and discrimination by patients, families, and visitors and association with burnout. *JAMA Netw Open*. 2022 May 2;5(5):e2213080. doi:10.1001/jamanetworkopen.2022.13080
3. Kane L. 'I cry but no one cares': physician burnout and depression report 2023. *Medscape*. January 27, 2023. Accessed October 14, 2023. https://www.medscape.com/slideshow/2023-lifestyle-burnout-6016058
4. Jolly S, Griffith KA, DeCastro R, et al. Gender differences in time spent on parenting and domestic responsibilities by high-achieving young physician-researchers. *Ann Int Med*. 2014;160(5):344–353. https://doi.org/10.7326/M13-0974

5. Jena AB, Olenski AR, Blumenthal DM. Sex differences in physician salary in US public medical schools. *JAMA Intern Med*. 2016;176(9):1294–1304. doi:10.1001/jamainternmed.2016.3284

6. Jena AB, Khullar D, Ho O, Olenski AR, Blumenthal DM. Sex differences in academic rank in US medical schools in 2014. *JAMA*. 2015 Sep 15;314(11):1149–58. doi:10.1001/jama.2015.10680

7. Martinez KA, Rothberg MB. Physician gender and its association with patient satisfaction and visit length: an observational study in telemedicine. *Cureus*. 2022 Sep 14;14(9):e29158. doi:10.7759/cureus.29158

8. Wallis CJD, Jerath A, Aminoltejari K, et al. Surgeon sex and long-term postoperative outcomes among patients undergoing common surgeries. *JAMA Surg*. 2023;158(11):1185–1194. doi:10.1001/jamasurg.2023.3744

9. Boyle P. The nation's medical schools grow more diverse. *Association of American Medical Colleges*. December 13, 2023. Accessed October 10, 2023. https://www.aamc.org/news/nation-s-medical-schools-grow-more-diverse

10. Desbiens NA, Vidaillet HJ Jr. Discrimination against international medical graduates in the United States residency program selection process. *BMC Med Educ*. 2010 Jan 25;10:5. doi:10.1186/1472-6920-10-5

11. Alsan M, Wanamaker M. Tuskegee and the health of black men. *Q J Econ*. 2018;133(1):407–455. doi:10.1093/qje/qjx029

12. James, CA, Bourgeois Florence T, Shannon MW. Association of race/ethnicity with emergency department wait times. *Pediatrics*. March 2005;115(3):e310–e315. https://doi.org/10.1542/peds.2004-1541

13. Schulman KA, Berlin JA, Harless W, et al. The effect of race and sex on physicians' recommendations for cardiac catheterization. *N Engl J Med*. 1999;340(8):618–626. doi:10.1056/NEJM199902253400806

14. Green CR, Anderson KO, Baker TA, et al. The unequal burden of pain: confronting racial and ethnic disparities in pain. *Pain Med*. 2003;4(3):277–294. https://doi.org/10.1046/j.1526-4637.2003.03034.x

15. Filut A, Alvarez M, Carnes M. Discrimination toward physicians of color: a systematic review. *J Natl Med Assoc*. 2020;112(2):117–140. doi:10.1016/j.jnma.2020.02.008

16. Takeshita J, Wang S, Loren AW, et al. Association of racial/ethnic and gender concordance between patients and physicians with patient experience ratings. *JAMA Netw Open*. 2020;3(11):e2024583. doi:10.1001/jamanetworkopen.2020.24583

17. Kane, L. Medscape physician compensation report 2023: your income vs your peers'. April 14, 2023. Accessed October 14, 2023. https://www.medscape.com/slideshow/2023-compensation-overview-6016341

5   Greed in Medicine

One of my favorite Olympic sports to watch is rowing. What intrigues me most is not only the strength and endurance required by team members to row at high speeds over a long distance, but how they move in synchrony to maximize the efficiency and effectiveness of their strokes. Rowers place their blades into the water at the same time and move their entire bodies in synchrony to generate maximum force when driving their blades through the water. In a quick and fluid motion, they simultaneously release their blades from the water and move them towards the bow of the boat to repeat the entire process.

Such harmony is essential for a rowing team to succeed. Failure to complete every component of the stroke at the same rate creates friction which slows down the boat.

In an ideal world, the healthcare system would operate like a well-tuned rowing team. Key stakeholders would work in harmony with the same goal in mind – putting the patient first. Pharmaceutical companies would be on the frontlines of innovation and prioritize the discovery of novel treatments at affordable prices to help as many people as possible. Insurance companies would look for creative ways to cover both preventative and life-sustaining treatments at reasonable rates. Healthcare administrators would be aligned with physicians and solely focused on helping them deliver the highest quality care. Hospitals would truly operate as not-for-profit entities and their leaders would be compensated accordingly. They would be more interested in addressing social determinants of health rather than adopting big business models to maximize profits. Earning a medical education would not be cost prohibitive which would help diversify the medical profession. The high cost of medical school is a reason why applicants are disproportionately white and of higher socioeconomic status (1). Tort reform would eliminate the urge to practice defensive medicine which leads to the ordering of unnecessary tests that patients are ultimately financially responsible for.

DOI: 10.4324/9781003473923-8

The benefits of an integrated, collaborative and synchronized healthcare system are too great to ignore. Uniting around a common, patient-centered vision would allow for a comprehensive and multifaceted emphasis on promoting wellness and eradicating illness with physicians leading the way. Such an approach would reduce inefficiencies that drive up the cost of healthcare. More importantly, such a cohesive system would benefit patients. They would have improved access to more affordable care.

Can you imagine how you would feel if you practiced medicine in such a system? You would actually feel proud to be part of a system that truly put the patient first. You would derive more fulfillment and meaning from your work because your sole focus would be on providing patients the best care possible. This is why you endured countless sacrifices to become a physician. Sure, practicing medicine is inherently emotionally taxing because of serving on the front lines of human suffering and being exposed to different forms of trauma. However, rates of physician burnout would be much lower if you had to contend with fewer systemic variables interfering with your ability to provide care. Your conscience would be much lighter if you did not hear stories from your patients about struggling to make ends meet due to the burden of medical bills or having delays in their care due to difficulties navigating a disjoined system.

The U.S. healthcare system has failed to put the patient first. Each member of the system is rowing in a different direction with money serving as their primary driving force. The financial self-interest of each sector has resulted in a fragmented system with individual profits taking precedence over patient care. Greed is the toxin that has eroded the values of empathy, compassion and integrity, which constitute the essence of medicine. You feel demoralized, defeated and disenchanted every time you observe compromises in patient care due to greedy tactics such as profiteering, price manipulation and revenue maximization (2). It shakes your moral compass and makes you question your decision to become a physician.

Let's explore how different parts of the healthcare system are prioritizing their own interests, often at the expense of patients.

Pharmaceuticals

Pharmaceuticals are a major expense in the U.S. healthcare system. In 2021, overall pharmaceutical expenditures totaled $576.9 billion, a 7.7% increase compared to 2020 (3). The high cost of prescription drugs threatens individual budgets. A poll from July 2023 showed that 25% of U.S. adults who take prescription medications reported difficulty affording them. This includes 40% of households with incomes less than $40,000 per year (4).

Pharmaceutical companies may justify high drug prices as essential for the development of novel drugs. However, higher drug prices have not translated into truly innovative treatments. Instead, pharmaceuticals have taken the financially safer path of making minor modifications to existing drugs with incremental improvements in efficacy or safety and raise their prices without constraint. The existence of monopolies and powerful lobbies which influence regulatory bodies allow them to engage in tactics that prioritize the financial gain of their shareholders. According to OpenSecrets, a nonpartisan, independent research group tracking money in U.S. politics, individual companies within the pharmaceuticals and health products sector spent over $381 million on lobbying in 2023 (5).

Changes to existing laws and regulations are essential to curb the current trends which put immense financial strain on patients and disrupt their care. Examples of measures to contain price spikes on pharmaceuticals include limiting the duration of patents, facilitating the approval process of generics, putting a cap on price increases and removing financial incentives for prescribing more expensive drugs (6).

Health Insurances

Health insurance companies have been raking in mammoth profits while insurance costs have soared. According to a Fierce Healthcare review of quarterly earnings reports, UnitedHealth Group led the way with $22.4 billion in profit for 2023, followed by CVS Health which made $8.3 billion in profit. Each company analyzed in the report increased their annual revenue (7).

It would be nice if insurance companies used some of their profits to provide patients with high-quality coverage at affordable rates. Unfortunately, this has not been the case. According to a 2022 poll by KFF, an independent source for health policy research, 48% of insured adults worry about affording their monthly health insurance premium. In addition, a significant portion of adults with employer-sponsored insurance and Marketplace coverage rate their insurance as "fair" or "poor" due to the cost of their monthly premiums or out-of-pocket costs to see a doctor (8).

In many cases, insurance companies request physicians to complete prior authorization which entails obtaining the insurance company's approval in advance that a prescribed treatment or medical service will be covered. This process allows the insurance company to determine coverage based on whether they deem an ordered exam or treatment to be medically necessary. In other words, prior authorization shifts medical decision-making from the treating physician to the insurance company even though it has never laid eyes on the patient.

Insurance companies contend that prior authorization curbs healthcare expenses by promoting cost-effective treatment options and preventing people from receiving unnecessary services. Unfortunately, this process has had the opposite effect because it is associated with higher overall utilization of healthcare resources, unnecessary waste and negative clinical outcomes. According to a 2022 survey by the American Medical Association, 94% of physicians reported that obtaining prior authorization was associated with delays in care. In addition, 89% of physicians reported that prior authorization requirements were associated with negative clinical outcomes. Furthermore, the majority of physicians reported that this process led to ineffective initial treatments and additional subsequent office visits. Finally, 33% of physicians reported that the use of prior authorization led to a serious, adverse event (9). Such results highlight the negative impact that this process has had on patients and the ability of physicians to care for them.

Hospitals

Starting in the 1960s, increased revenue from the advent of Medicare and greater insurance coverage influenced hospitals to adopt business practices. Some hospitals even changed their mission statements to emphasize the importance of financial considerations (10).

In keeping up with business practices, hospitals have had an explosion in administrators. A typical U.S. services industry has approximately 0.85 administrative workers for each person in a specialized role. However, the U.S. healthcare system has twice as many administrative workers as physicians and nurses. There were an estimated 5.4 million administrative employees in 2017, with over 1 million added since 2001 (11).

Here is another figure to illustrate the disproportionate increase in hospital administrators. The number of physicians in the United States grew by 150% between 1975 and 2010, an increase consistent with the rate of population growth. During that same time period, the number of healthcare administrators increased by 3,200% (11).

Some would say the growing number of administrators was necessary to keep pace with changes in the healthcare industry. My experience is the increase has been excessive resulting in redundancy and division within the healthcare system. As a personal example, my employer audits physician charts on a yearly basis to ensure we are following proper documentation and coding practices. This is a prudent practice which I fully support because it educates physicians on these important topics and deters fraudulent activity. When I first joined my employer about a decade ago, I would meet with one or two auditors to go over the audit results. In 2023, the meeting consisted of three auditors, two practice managers and a physician leader with an administrative role. As a physician who has a decade of experience with the same employer, did I need to meet with six administrators to be told that I passed my annual audit? I will let you be the judge.

Most troubling is that administrative decisions can compromise patient care. Published in the *New England Journal of Medicine,* Dr. O'Donnell shares how the administrative decision to discontinue a two-decade hospital smoking cessation program negatively impacted patient care (12). Administrative decisions can unintentionally lead to breaches in care because they are often made by people who have never practiced clinical medicine and are myopically focused on cost-savings. As physicians, we experience moral injury every time we bear witness to such outcomes.

Another result of adopting big business practices has been the disproportionate rise in compensation for healthcare executives who often have salaries and benefits in the millions of dollars. Their rise in compensation has mirrored the climb in CEO wages across corporate America. The wide disparity in compensation for CEOs at nonprofit hospitals compared to nonprofit entities outside medicine highlights how hospitals have shifted away from their roots and towards a more corporate model. In 2018, the average annual CEO pay in most nonprofit industries ranged between $100,000 and $200,000. Hospital CEOs often make ten times that amount (10).

Tactics employed to extract payments from patients, even those with low incomes, further exemplify how hospitals have become indistinguishable from for-profit businesses and relentless in their mission to maximize profits. A *New York Times* investigation revealed that staff members of a nonprofit hospital were instructed on how to approach patients and pressure them to pay their bills. If patients did not pay, they were sent to debt collectors who only intensified the pressure (13).

An additional tactic employed by hospitals to boost profits involves the lack of price transparency for hospital services. Can you imagine shopping for groceries or ordering from a restaurant menu that did not list prices? You would have a hard time sticking to a budget and often overpay for goods. This is exactly what is transpiring in healthcare where unsuspecting patients, often in desperate need of medical care, blindly trust the system to operate in their best interest. Being an educated consumer is nearly impossible when your health depends on navigating a fragmented system that lacks transparency. As a result, patients accept services without being fully informed upfront of their cost. Expanded price transparency would curb healthcare expenditures by helping employers be more informed when purchasing health benefits for their workers. It would also allow regulators to more effectively monitor healthcare market competition, ensuring patients have access to lower-cost, high-quality care (14).

These tactics illustrate how hospitals have lost their moral compass. They have diverged from their roots of putting the patient first. Instead, they view patients as a revenue source to meet their financial goals. It is one thing for the pharmaceutical and health insurance industries to develop a gluttony for profitability. However, hospitals following suit is undeniable proof that the U.S. healthcare has fallen into a dire existential crisis which requires radical restructuring of the system from the ground up.

The Bottom Line

Research shows that doing things in synchrony can strengthen social ties and create a greater sense of well-being. Interpersonal synchrony promotes predictability in complex dynamic environments, facilitates information flow, reduces working memory load and builds greater group cohesion (15).

Unfortunately, you are immersed in a disjointed system that completely lacks synchrony because everyone is rowing in a different direction. There is a lack of information flow because the different components of the system work in silos and do not communicate effectively with each other. Due to their lack of clinical knowledge, hospital administrators fail to appreciate how top-down decisions negatively impact patient care and your ability to provide it. There is a lack of predictability in your workflow because policies and initiatives that are periodically introduced by hospital leadership abruptly shift your focus onto different targets.

During a patient encounter, not only are you trying to solve a patient's health concern, but also trying to simultaneously meet the hospital's latest initiative. Don't forget to screen your patients for [*fill in the blank*] so the hospital can bill for it, even though it is irrelevant to the visit. Never mind this is an established, well-known patient who is visiting you for a specific problem and you have a limited amount of time to address it. Even if well intended, administrative initiatives add unnecessary friction and redundancy to your work flow, which takes a toll on your working memory and emotions.

Not only is there a lack of synchrony, but persistent tension and conflict because you have to protect patients from the same parties that are supposed to care for them. You have to advocate for your patients every time an insurance company refuses to cover a prescribed treatment. A part of you dies inside every time someone undermines your efforts due to their self-serving interests.

How can you not suffer from burnout and moral injury being part of such a broken system? How can you not be irate with what is transpiring? Medicine was a calling. You entered medicine with the purest intentions and made tremendous sacrifices to become a physician, only to have the system rip away your life's passion because they want to make a profit from people in their most vulnerable time. You can endure only so many blows before you are completely wounded and burned out.

Key stakeholders of the healthcare system do not share your mission. Once you see this truth, you cannot unsee it. Coming to this realization is painful but also liberating. Now that you see what is transpiring, you can better justify setting firm boundaries. If they view patients as a revenue source, what makes you think they view you any differently? You are also a revenue source whose purpose is to generate the system as much money as possible. This is a dehumanizing process and the complete antithesis of what medicine should stand for. Due to their insatiable appetite for profits, they work you to the extreme. The only difference is that you have more authority, autonomy and leverage than your patients. You can fight back because you are the expert with the abilities, skills and qualifications to thrive and earn a living in a variety of settings.

Ignoring the realities of how the healthcare system operates will not make them go away. Such an approach only makes you more vulnerable to exploitation. You need to keep your guard up and defend yourself from attempts to exploit you. This is a matter of self-preservation. Carrying this guard is exhausting and makes it exponentially harder to serve your patients. It would be so much more pleasant if you did not have to be guarded because everyone in healthcare worked together for the common mission of putting the patient first. Unfortunately, you do not have this luxury. Radical change is necessary for healthcare to return to its noble roots. In the meantime, your best option is to advocate for yourself and your patients because greed has tainted medicine.

References

1. Millo L, Ho N, Ubel PA. The cost of applying to medical school – a barrier to diversifying the profession. *NEJM.* 2019 Oct 16;381(16):1505–1508. doi:10.1056/NEJMp1906704
2. Berwick DM. *Salve lucrum:* the existential threat of greed in US health care. *JAMA.* 2023;329(8):629–630. doi:10.1001/jama.2023.0846
3. Tichy EM, Hoffman JM, Suda KJ, et al. National trends in prescription drug expenditures and projections for 2022. *Am J Health Syst Pharm.* 2022;79(14):1158–1172. doi:10.1093/ajhp/zxac102
4. Wager E, Telesford I, Cox C, Amin K. What are the recent and forecasted trends in prescription drug spending? Peterson-KFF Health System Tracker. September 15, 2023. Accessed April 20, 2024. https://www.healthsystemtracker.org/chart-collection/recent-forecasted-trends-prescription-drug-spending/#item-perc ent-of-total-rx-spending-by-oop-private-insurance-and-medicare_nhe-projecti ons-2018-27
5. Open Secrets. Industry profile: pharmaceuticals/health products. Accessed April 23, 2024. https://www.opensecrets.org/federal-lobbying/industries/summ ary?cycle=2023&id=H04
6. Rajkumar SV. The high cost of prescription drugs: causes and solutions. *Blood Cancer J.* 2020 Jun 23;10(6):71. doi:10.1038/s41408-020-0338-x
7. Minemyer P. Medicare Advantage headwinds didn't prevent payers from turning a profit in 2023. *Fierce Healthcare.* February 9, 2024. Accessed April 23, 2024. https://www.fiercehealthcare.com/payers/medicare-advantage-headwinds-didnt-prevent-payers-turning-profit-2023

8. Lopes L, Montero A, Presiado M, Hamel L. Americans' challenges with health care costs. *KFF*. March 1, 2024. Accessed April 23, 2024. https://www.kff.org/health-costs/issue-brief/americans-challenges-with-health-care-costs/

9. 2022 AMA prior authorization (PA) physician survey. *AMA*. March 13, 2023. Accessed April 23, 2024. https://www.ama-assn.org/system/files/prior-authorization-survey.pdf

10. Saini V, Garber J, Brownlee S. Nonprofit hospital CEO compensation: how much is enough. *Health Affairs*. February 10, 2022. Accessed April 26, 2024. https://www.healthaffairs.org/content/forefront/nonprofit-hospital-ceo-compensation-much-enough

11. Cantlupe J. The rise (and rise) of the healthcare administrator. *Athenainsight*. November 7, 2017. Accessed April 24, 2024. https://www.athenahealth.com/knowledge-hub/sites/insight/files/The%20rise%20%28and%20rise%29%20of%20the%20healthcare%20administrator.pdf

12. O'Donnell WJ. Reducing administrative harm in medicine – clinicians and administrators together. *N Engl J Med*. 2022;386(25):2429–2432. doi:10.1056/NEJMms2202174

13. Silver-Greenberg J, Thomas K. They were entitled to free care. Hospitals hounded them to pay. September 24, 2022. Updated December 15, 2022. Accessed April 28, 2024. *The New York Times*. https://www.nytimes.com/2022/09/24/business/nonprofit-hospitals-poor-patients.html

14. Whaley CM, Perkins J, Bai Ge. Congress has the opportunity to deliver health care price transparency. *Health Affairs*. March 18, 2024. Accessed April 28, 2024. https://www.healthaffairs.org/content/forefront/congress-has-opportunity-deliver-health-care-price-transparency-american-people

15. Hoehl S, Fairhurst M, Schirmer A. Interactional synchrony: signals, mechanisms and benefits. *Soc Cogn Affect Neurosci*. 2021;16(1–2):5–18. doi:10.1093/scan/nsaa024

6   Secrecy in Medicine

Imagine a work colleague is going through a hard time. You can see it in their eyes and body language that something is bothering them. There has been a change in their demeanor. They have started coming in late to work and appear disengaged. They have been quieter than usual and keeping to themselves. They even uncharacteristically lost their temper and raised their voice at staff over a minor scheduling blunder. You naturally check on them out of concern. They say they don't want to talk about it and insist they're ok, even though they're clearly not. You tell them to reach out should they need anything. They politely thank you but never take the offer.

How would you feel about this scenario? Odds are the change in their behavior would leave you feeling uneasy and concerned. You might wonder about what is troubling them and whether they have the necessary support to overcome it. You might also be concerned about how things will ultimately play out if they don't get the help they need.

Your concerns would be warranted because you don't know what your colleague is going through and have no evidence that there is a plan in place to overcome their troubles. You would have felt more reassured if they had replied in the following manner:

> I am dealing with a problem at work and have expressed my concerns to our practice manager and department chair. It really bothers me that my schedule is double booked without consulting with me first. I hope this situation is resolved because it compromises my ability to provide quality patient care. Regardless, I have updated my resume and started exploring my options just in case the work situation does not improve.

You would find such a response more reassuring because your colleague is not in denial about their situation. They are acknowledging the existence of a problem and have set a plan in motion to address it. This tells you that

DOI: 10.4324/9781003473923-9

their situation will improve one way or another. Either the stressor contributing to their troubles will be addressed or they will circumvent it by changing their work environment.

Unfortunately, such responses are not common among physicians. Our reflex is to bottle up our thoughts and feelings about stressors without seeking any help to address them. According to the 2024 Medscape Report on Physician Burnout and Depression, 71% of respondents have suffered from burnout for at least 13 months, and 42% have suffered for over two years. Yet, only 33% would feel comfortable opening dialogue with coworkers about seeking help from burnout. What is more astonishing is that 53% of respondents reported they had never sought professional help for their burnout and depression in the past, nor would they seek out such help in the future (1).

Take a moment to consider the significance of this data. This study of 9,226 U.S. physicians from 29 different specialties reveals that the majority do not feel comfortable even having a conversation about their emotional difficulties, let alone seek help to address them. Instead, they cope by putting up a shield to conceal their suffering. They show up, day after day, and care for patients while suffering tremendously behind the disguise of a brave, stoic face. They endure the effects of burnout for years until the pain becomes unbearable.

Imagine if our patients adopted such an approach for their health issues. What if they did not want professional help to manage their hypertension or diabetes but insisted on dealing with these conditions on their own or completely ignored them? What do you think would be the ultimate outcome of their approach? It would not be good. Not taking the proper course of action to address a problem only makes it exponentially harder to tackle.

From a clinical standpoint, you are aware of this reality. Intervening early in the disease process can spare future complications. Keeping your routine colonoscopy to remove a few polyps can prevent them from turning into cancerous which would require more invasive medical interventions. Making lifestyle modifications at the earliest signs of prediabetes is preferable to waiting until the condition has evolved into full-blown diabetes. Waiting to intervene not only makes it harder to contain the underlying condition. It also requires more radical interventions because you have a number of complications to contend with.

Your mental health is no different. Delaying help for depression or burnout allows these conditions to grow in severity and wreak havoc on your physical, mental and social health. It has been shown that delays in the treatment of depression result in worst outcomes (2). With every passing day that you delay seeking help, you are digging a deeper hole that becomes harder to climb out of.

Ironically, as physicians, this is how we respond to our emotional diffi-culties. We endure pain for years without revealing any signs of suffering, even to those who are closest to us. This approach allows for the emotional pain to intensify and have a greater impact. It is remarkable that we can endure pain for years without any help, while consistently showing up to fulfill work, family and social responsibilities. The fact that you have walked this path, all alone, is undeniable proof of how resilient you truly are.

However, you are resilient to a fault. This is not the correct approach to address burnout or any other emotional difficulty. You know this because you would never recommend such an approach to any patient or loved one. You would never advise anyone to bear their physical or mental health problems on their own. You would encourage them to get the help they need.

So, why the double standard? Why do you not give yourself permission to practice what you preach?

The truth is a number of factors keep you, and countless physicians, from seeking help and support, especially when you need it the most. Let's explore how these factors influence you to stay silent during difficult times in your life.

Stigma against Mental Health

A major reason you do not seek help for burnout, depression or any other emotional difficulty is because the culture of medicine has perpetuated the stigma against mental health. You fear that such difficulties would be seen as a sign of weakness or lack of clinical competence, which would sub-sequently compromise your professional reputation and opportunities for career advancement. Hence, you hide your suffering like the rest of your colleagues – behind a façade consisting of a white coat, fancy degrees hanging from your office walls and prestigious titles.

The 2024 Medscape Report on Physician Burnout and Depression reveals the magnitude of the stigma. When asked about the reasons for not telling anyone about their depression, 21% of physicians considered depression to be a weakness, 37% that people would think less of them and 44% that people would doubt their clinical abilities (1).

I find it concerning that so many physicians consider depression to be a weakness, when it is a health condition that requires treatment, the nature of which is determined by the etiology, symptomatology and severity of the condition. Despite our medical knowledge, we view mental health conditions as character defects to be ashamed of and treat them differently than physical health conditions. You would never feel ashamed to seek treatment for a broken bone, abdominal pain or a concerning skin lesion. The same cannot be said for mental health difficulties.

If trained medical professionals view depression as a character defect, you can imagine the views of people without any medical training. Why would they seek mental health treatment when their own healthcare providers consider it a sign of weakness? More work needs to be done to eradicate the stigma against mental health in medicine and society. We also need to have more compassion for anyone suffering from mental health difficulties. They are not only combating the debilitating symptoms of their condition but also the stigma associated with it.

Repercussions from State Medical Boards

Another reason physicians suffer in silence is the fear that seeking mental healthcare can compromise their medical license and ability to practice medicine. 42% of respondents in the 2024 Medscape Report on Physician Burnout and Depression reported not telling anyone about their depression for fear that their state medical board or employer might find out (1). Another study of 5,829 physicians found that nearly 40% of respondents would be reluctant to seek formal treatment of a mental health condition due to a fear of repercussions on their medical licensure (3).

Many state medical boards ask physicians about prior mental health conditions or treatment on license applications. Such questions prevent physicians from seeking professional mental healthcare due to a fear of compromising their license. This fear is understandable as there are documented cases of physicians facing scrutiny, even disciplinary action, after revealing past treatment. An Oregon emergency department physician reported that informing her state medical board about a previous episode of mania resulted in public disclosures of her condition, a four-month long investigation, lost income and a tarnished reputation at work (4).

Questioning physicians about their mental health history does not protect patients from clinicians who may not be fit to provide care. Prior mental health difficulties have no reflection on a physician's current ability to care for patients. On the contrary, these questions have a paradoxically harmful effect on both patients and physicians. By serving as barriers to mental healthcare, they discourage physicians from addressing any emotional difficulties that could compromise their ability to practice medicine. State medical boards and employers should encourage physicians to prioritize their mental health and facilitate access to care. Such measures would help physicians be better equipped to handle the rigorous demands of clinical medicine.

This perspective is supported by governing bodies as they do not require credentialing and licensure organizations to ask physicians about prior mental health history on applications. In particular, the Joint Commission encourages organizations to limit inquiries to conditions that currently impair a clinician's ability to perform their job (5).

On a positive note, there appears to be a major culture shift in overcoming this barrier to care. According to Medscape, physicians in 21 states are no longer being asked by medical boards about their mental health or substance use history during license applications (6).

Adverse Patient Outcomes

Patient safety incidents are common in the U.S. healthcare system. According to a report published in the BMJ, medical error is the third leading cause of death in the United States, after heart disease and cancer, accounting for more than 250,000 deaths per year (7). Systemic factors create conditions that make physicians prone to errors in the workplace. Having a schedule crammed with patients while documenting on a cumbersome electronic medical record and simultaneously responding to electronic messages from patients can make even the most competent physician prone to error. Organizations need to take measures to address the working conditions contributing to them.

Despite the multifactorial nature of adverse events, they have a profound psychological impact on physicians. A systematic review and meta-analysis of 11,649 healthcare providers found that the majority experienced troubling memories, anxiety, anger with themselves, remorse, fear of future errors, embarrassment and guilt in the aftermath of an adverse event (8).

Such responses are completely understandable. We deeply care about the quality of our work and the patients we serve. The thought that someone could be harmed under our care is a disturbing experience that shakes us to our core. It is common for physicians to doubt their professional skills, consider a career change or even leave the profession altogether after an adverse patient outcome.

Despite their emotional toll, physicians often suffer in silence following an adverse patient outcome. There is also a perceived lack of organizational support. A survey studying the emotional impact of medical errors on practicing physicians in the U.S. and Canada found that only 10% of respondents felt their healthcare organizations supported them adequately in coping with error-related stress (9).

I have even seen cases in which physicians were disparaged by colleagues following an adverse patient outcome. Morbidity and Mortality (M&M) conferences are an Accreditation Council for Graduate Medical Education (ACGME) mandated educational series that occur at institutions with residency training programs. The objective of this conference is to provide an opportunity for faculty and trainees to explore the management details of clinical cases in which morbidity or mortality occurred (10).

A physician described to me how colleagues publicly attacked them at an M&M conference for their treatment choices, but privately told them afterwards that they would have taken a similar approach. They used the forum as an opportunity to elevate themselves by disparaging this physician.

Medical Malpractice

Litigation is a fairly common experience in medicine. An analysis of malpractice data for physicians covered by a large professional liability insurer found that 7.4% of them had a malpractice claim for each year of the study period (11).

Going through litigation is an emotionally challenging experience. As physicians, our identity is deeply connected to the quality of our work. A malpractice suit that alleges medical negligence or wrongdoing is an existential threat to your sense of self. A survey administered to physicians with both open and closed claims found that 56% of them had experienced a psychological reaction to the claim. Many also acknowledged that the claims impacted how they practiced medicine. They subsequently took more defensive measures by ordering additional tests for medical workups and avoiding patients they considered higher risk (12).

Going through a medical malpractice claim can even take a toll on a physician's health. There are documented cases of catastrophic vascular complications that occurred to otherwise healthy physicians immediately prior to or during the trial phase of medical malpractice litigations (13).

Considering the enormous toll of malpractice suits on a physician's mental and physical health, it is unfortunate they have to suffer in silence when facing them. Legal counsel advises defendants not to discuss details of a case with anyone due to concerns of saying something that could jeopardize their defense. However, this approach can exacerbate feelings of isolation and self-doubt during an emotionally challenging time.

The Culture of Medicine

As discussed in chapter 3, exposure to traumatic events is common in medicine. Instead of cultivating a safe environment to explore and process one's thoughts and feelings behind emotionally difficult clinical cases, medicine has trained you to be self-reliant and stoic. You are used to suppressing your feelings as you automatically move from one clinical encounter to the next. Though useful in a variety of clinical settings, this approach also comes with pitfalls.

When taken to the extreme, self-reliance can be a barrier to help-seeking behavior (14). Seeking help requires you to be vulnerable and rely on someone else for support and guidance. This process can be hard because you are used to being the expert with the final say in decision making. As a result, you are more likely to stay silent and rely on your own abilities to overcome difficulties.

Stoicism is an additional barrier to processing your thoughts and feelings. According to the Stoics, the ideal agent has no emotions because they are considered barriers to reason. The aim is not moderation, but rather a life without emotions (15).

The problem with stoic ideology is that it neglects the important role emotions play in your life. They are rich sources of data that can guide your decisions. You have a right to feel angry when you encounter injustice. It is ok to feel betrayed because medicine has not turned into the career you had envisioned. You have a right to feel anxious going into work because you are so busy it feels like drinking water from a firehose. Your emotions are valid and a signal to pay close attention to. They are trying to convey information and will not subside until you take the proper course of action to address the matter at hand.

From this perspective, suppressing your thoughts and feelings is not a wise long-term strategy because you are discarding valuable information. Furthermore, evidence shows that suppression can paradoxically intensify the unwanted thoughts and feelings you are trying to avoid (16).

A healthier approach is to cultivate self-awareness. Learn to identify what you are thinking and feeling. The ability to hold space and pay attention to your emotions, even if they are uncomfortable, will help you better decipher what they are trying to convey.

The Outcome

Sharing your thoughts and feelings is not in your DNA. Nor is asking for help and support. Medicine has trained you to keep your suffering a secret. You learned this early in your training as you put on a brave face to survive the grueling demands of medical school and residency. To this day, you rely on the same defense mechanism. You put on the same brave face for patients, colleagues and loved ones. However, this is a façade. Hidden behind it is great pain, anguish and desperation.

The only difference is you are carrying even greater pain and anguish compared to the earlier stages of your career. When you were younger, you held out hope that life would be better upon completing your training and becoming an attending physician. You believed that having more income, autonomy and authority would translate into a fulfilling career.

Unfortunately, this has not been the case. That ray of hope was a mirage that has been engulfed by a cloud of desperation. Your goal is to leave medicine by either saving enough money to retire early or finding an alternative, non-clinical source of income. You are not alone in this pursuit.

Despite the demands of practicing clinical medicine, many physicians are investing their scarce time and energy to take on additional work outside medicine. A survey found that 39% of physicians had a side gig and devoted over 20 hours per month to it. The majority conceded that earning extra money was the main motivator behind their side gig (17).

The fact that so many physicians are looking to reduce their financial dependence on medicine is evidence of how unbearable it has become. Their solution to the burnout riddle is working even more hours with the hopes of finding a revenue source to replace medicine. This strategy is also a mirage and bound to fail for most. The vast majority of these endeavors are not generating the extra money that physicians had hoped for (17).

The suffering among physicians is widespread and pervasive. Yet, instead of addressing the root of the problem, we double down on familiar behaviors and work even harder. We take on second jobs that often do not pay enough to be worth our time. This is a flawed strategy that only exacerbates the intensity of your burnout.

A Healthier Approach

The solution to burnout is not to work harder or make more money. The solution is to acknowledge your emotional difficulties and seek the help your need. Instead of suppressing your thoughts and feelings, share them in a safe space with a trained professional. This will provide you with necessary insights and strategies to tackle stressors impacting your life.

We need to fight against mental health stigma by having the courage to share our emotional experiences and support colleagues facing adversity. Isolation exacerbates suffering because it serves as fertile ground for shame to get a hold of you and grow without restraint. This creates the illusion that there is something fundamentally wrong with you because you feel like the only one suffering. Sharing your experience in a safe space is a powerful reminder you are not alone. The majority of physicians are suffering because of a number of systemic factors. They are the primary drivers of your emotional difficulties.

There is a misconception that enduring pain is a sign of resilience. In other words, the more pain you can endure in silence, the more resilient you are. In reality, resilience has nothing to do with how you carry your pain. You don't have to prove your resilience to anyone. The fact that you have made it this far in your medical career is undeniable proof of your resilience.

Nor is your pain a sign of weakness. Your pain is valid and justified. It is a signal that medicine has lost its soul. Systemic factors that prioritize profits over patient care are interfering with your ability to practice medicine. How can you not be hurt by what is transpiring?

Seek support sooner than later. As stoic, self-reliant perfectionists, we have a tendency of staying silent until there is a crisis and are at the point of no return. Certainly, reach out for help if you are in a dire situation. However, do not wait until the final hour to seek help. Make your mental health a priority early and often. Reach out at the earliest signs of distress. Examples include an increase in anxiety and irritability, not enjoying activities you typically enjoy, having sleep difficulties or wanting an alcoholic beverage to unwind at night. These early signs are cracks in your psychological armor and need to be addressed before bigger problems arise.

Finally, if you are reluctant to seek help, do it with a loved one in mind. This could be a family member, partner, friend or colleague. You do not live in a bubble. Seeking help will greatly benefit the people who matter most to you. Becoming a better version of yourself will allow you to be more engaged and present with them. It will also benefit countless colleagues who keep their suffering a secret. Your actions are a blueprint that give them permission to break free from the shackles of secrecy and reach out for help.

References

1. McKenna J. Medscape physician burnout and depression report 2024: 'we have much work to do.' *Medscape*. January 26, 2024. Accessed May 20, 2024.
2. Ghio L, Gotelli S, Marcenaro M, Amore M, Natta W. Duration of untreated illness and outcomes in unipolar depression: a systematic review and meta-analysis. *J Affect Disord*. 2014;152–154:45–51. doi:10.1016/j.jad.2013.10.002
3. Dyrbye LN, West CP, Sinsky CA, Goeders LE, Satele DV, Shanafelt TD. Medical licensure questions and physician reluctance to seek care for mental health conditions. *Mayo Clin Proc*. 2017;92(10):1486–1493. doi:10.1016/j.mayocp.2017.06.020
4. Lehmann C. An MD's nightmare began with reporting her manic episode to the medical board. *Medscape*. November 3, 2021. Accessed May 26, 2024.
5. The Joint Commission. The Joint Commission statement on health care worker mental health. 2021. Accessed May 26, 2024. https://www.jointcommission.org/resources/patient-safety-topics/healthcare-workforce-safety-and-well-being/resources-from-the-joint-commission/
6. Lehmann C. Mental health questions cut from MD licensing applications in 21 states. *Medscape*. July 10, 2023. Accessed May 26, 2024. https://www.medscape.com/viewarticle/994163
7. Makary MA, Daniel M. Medical error-the third leading cause of death in the US. *BMJ*. 2016;353:i2139. doi:https://doi.org/10.1136/bmj.i2139
8. Busch IM, Moretti F, Purgato M, Barbui C, Wu AW, Rimondini M. Psychological and psychosomatic symptoms of second victims of adverse events: a systematic review and meta-analysis [published correction appears in *J Patient Saf*. 2020 Sep;16(3):e211. doi:10.1097/PTS.0000000000000779]. *J Patient Saf*. 2020;16(2):e61–e74. doi:10.1097/PTS.0000000000000589

9. Waterman AD, Garbutt J, Hazel E, et al. The emotional impact of medical errors on practicing physicians in the United States and Canada. *Jt Comm J Qual Patient Saf.* 2007;33(8):467–476. doi:10.1016/s1553-7250(07)33050-x

10. Kravet SJ, Howell E, Wright SM. Morbidity and mortality conference, grand rounds, and the ACGME's core competencies. *J Gen Intern Med.* 2006;21(11):1192–1194. doi:10.1111/j.1525-1497.2006.00523.x

11. Jena AB, Seabury S, Lakdawalla D, Chandra A. Malpractice risk according to physician specialty. *N Engl J Med.* 2011;365(7):629–636. doi:10.1056/NEJMsa1012370

12. Vizcaíno-Rakosnik M, Martin-Fumadó C, Arimany-Manso J, Gómez-Durán EL. The impact of malpractice claims on physicians' well-being and practice. *J Patient Saf.* 2022;18(1):46–51. doi:10.1097/PTS.0000000000000800

13. Maroon JC. Catastrophic cardiovascular complications from medical malpractice stress syndrome. *J Neurosurg.* 2019 Mar 29;130(6):2081–2085. doi:10.3171/2019.1.JNS183622

14. Ishikawa A, Rickwood D, Bariola E, Bhullar N. Autonomy versus support: self-reliance and help-seeking for mental health problems in young people. *Soc Psychiatry Psychiatr Epidemiol.* 2023;58(3):489–499. doi:10.1007/s00127-022-02361-4

15. Stanford Encyclopedia of Philosophy. October 7, 2007. Revised February 13, 2024. Accessed May 28, 2024. https://plato.stanford.edu/entries/seneca/#TheEmo

16. Wenzlaff RM, Wegner DM. Thought suppression. *Annu Rev Psychol.* 2000;51:59–91. doi:10.1146/annurev.psych.51.1.59

17. McKenna J. What you love or loathe in your side hustle: Medscape physician side gigs report 2023. *Medscape.* October 12, 2023. Accessed June 1, 2024.

Part 3
A Path to a Better Self

7 Make Yourself a Priority

The following scenario is all too familiar. A patient presents with a chief complaint of fatigue. They describe a hectic schedule filled with work and home responsibilities. They report having no time for self-care. They are too busy to find time for leisure or exercise. Their only break comes from staying up late to enjoy a couple nightcaps before going to bed.

Getting out of bed in the mornings has been a challenge. They hit the snooze button multiple times before they finally get their day started. All morning, they dread going into work where morale has been low due to being short staffed and overworked. Unfortunately, things have not been better at home due to escalating tensions with their partner.

They report consuming multiple cups of coffee and energy drinks throughout the day to combat high levels of fatigue. Consuming caffeine also improves their concentration which has been low. They inquire about a workup to determine the underlying cause of their symptoms and treatment options to improve their energy and focus.

The answer to this clinical scenario is fairly obvious for even the most novice physician. Being under high levels of chronic stress is exhausting. You would order blood work to be thorough and rule out underlying causes of their presentation. However, you would also educate your patient on the negative impact of chronic stress on their energy and concentration. You would encourage them to make their health a priority by allocating more time for physical activity and sleep. You would also counsel them to cut back on their caffeine intake because it interferes with sleep onset. Finally, you would educate them on the health risks of daily alcohol use. A number of psychosocial factors are contributing to their presentation. Addressing them is essential to improve their symptoms.

It is easy to notice when others have veered off track and offer them advice to course correct. However, it is much more difficult to detect when we have drifted off course, because we are not always objective with ourselves. Defense mechanisms, such as denial, rationalization and

DOI: 10.4324/9781003473923-11

intellectualization cloud our self-assessment. We subconsciously fall for unhealthy habits without fully understanding their long-term impact on us and those around us.

Truth is we are no different than our patients. We might have a greater depth of knowledge about how the body functions. We have been trained to diagnose and treat different health conditions. However, being physicians does not make us exempt from the struggles of the human condition. We grapple with the same vices as everyone else.

Knowledge does not equate wisdom. It is one thing to counsel your patients on the damaging effects of alcohol use, binge eating and a sedentary lifestyle. It is another to practice what you preach. A national survey of over 9,100 physicians showed that 32% of respondents cope with burnout by eating junk food, 22% by drinking alcohol and 18% by binge eating. In addition, 2% reported smoking cigarettes and another 2% using cannabis products (1). Evidence shows that occupational distress increases the odds of engaging in problematic alcohol use and binge eating (2).

On a cognitive level, you know the difference between healthy and unhealthy habits. You do not need a medical degree to know that eating junk food, drinking alcohol and binge eating is not good for your health. You also know exercise, healthy eating habits, meditation, journaling, spending time with loved ones and getting adequate sleep are beneficial for your physical and mental health. Despite this knowledge, it is hard to stick with healthy habits. The same national survey of 9,100 physicians showed that only 50% of them cope with burnout by exercise, 45% by talking to family or friends and 22% by meditating (1).

Sticking with healthy habits is difficult for a number of reasons. First of all, they take effort. Mustering energy for exercise, journaling or meditation can feel insurmountable when you are depleted due to burnout or depression. In addition, these strategies do not yield immediate benefits. You will not experience the euphoria of a runner's high a few minutes into your jog. Nor will you have a sense of inner peace after your first meditation session. On the contrary, you are more likely to experience an initial spike in discomfort, frustration and anxiety while pushing your body and mind through unfamiliar territory.

It is human nature to pursue the path of least resistance. If you do not intentionally and consistently engage in healthy practices, you will automatically fall for unhealthy ones. Problematic behaviors such as alcohol and substance use, eating junk food and excessive screen time will fill the void because they require little effort to have an immediate impact on your emotional state. Their mind-numbing properties instantly quell feelings of irritability, sadness or anxiety.

Considering this benefit, you may ask what's the harm in having a nightcap, a smoke or extra screen time if it is not happening at work or interfering with your ability to care for patients. After all, you are a physician and worked hard all day. You treat patients who have it far worse than you.

This mindset is an example of your defense mechanisms at work. Denial and rationalization minimize the risks associated with these behaviors. Their rapid onset but brief duration of action makes them highly addictive. Over time, you build tolerance and require greater quantities to obtain the same relief. One drink at night turns into two or three. A hit turns into the entire joint. Thirty minutes of screen time turns into a four-hour Netflix binge that keeps you up later than anticipated. You are playing with fire when relying on these behaviors.

In addition, unhealthy habits come with emotional baggage. It only a matter of time before the brief emotional bliss is replaced by the toxic effects of shame which shatters your relationship with yourself. If you could put down your emotional guard and be honest with yourself, you would acknowledge that you do not feel good about yourself when you engage in these behaviors because you know they are not good for you. They ultimately come at a cost to your physical, mental and social health. You would never recommend that a patient or loved one engages in them to cope with their reality. Why are you exempt from this truth?

Unhealthy behaviors take you away from loved ones. You think about having a drink or smoke more than you care to admit. You look forward to it at the end of a hard day. Precious time with loved ones feels like a chore that stands in the way of what you crave most – going to your familiar place to engage in your familiar behavior to numb your thoughts and feelings.

Others having it worse is not an excuse to continue your behavior. Not currently meeting criteria for an alcohol use, substance use or eating disorder does not mean your behavior is not problematic. You are flying a plane on a downward trajectory. It is only a matter of time before everything comes crashing down.

The ancient Greeks had a saying "νους υγιής εν σώματι υγιεί" meaning a healthy mind in a healthy body. It is essential that you make yourself a priority by allocating time for healthy habits that promote your physical and mental health. If you do not commit to this process, unhealthy vices will automatically fill the void. Life is hard and we all have to cope with our realities. The question is whether you intentionally rely on healthy strategies or mindlessly fall for unhealthy ones.

Though they require more initial effort and energy, healthy habits do not come with baggage. You do not have to hide them from others. Nor do you spiral into shame after engaging in them. Instead, these behaviors build your self-esteem. You feel better about who you are and who you are becoming after exercising, meditating or making a healthy meal. Healthy behaviors help you become a better version of yourself and reach your fullest potential.

Prioritizing your health is not a panacea. It will not solve the systemic factors that plague medicine and interfere with your ability to provide patient care. These factors are the primary drivers of burnout. However, it will limit their impact on you. You cannot simply abandon your health and engage in unhealthy habits just because medicine has not turned into the career you had envisioned. This only makes a bad situation worse by further hindering your ability to serve your family, patients and community at the highest level.

Developing daily healthy habits will help you be better equipped to rise above the broken healthcare system that is contributing to your burnout. I will present seven practices to promote your physical, mental and social health with tips on how to make them an integral part of your life.

One final note before diving into them. As physicians, we have a tendency of trying to achieve too much too soon. A part of you will want to make radical changes and incorporate every practice in your hectic schedule. This approach can make the process of prioritizing your health overwhelming and exponentially harder to make any positive change. A healthier approach is to focus on incorporating a single healthy practice in your busy schedule. Pick a behavior you would find enjoyable and stick with it. Give it time to become integrated into your identity by practicing it consistently. Once you have mastered it and are reaping its benefits, consider incorporating the next practice.

Exercise

The benefits of exercise for physical health are well documented. However, exercise is also beneficial for your overall mood and anxiety because it reduces sympathetic nervous system and hypothalamic-pituitary-adrenal axis reactivity, increases serotonin and brain-derived neurotrophic factor and positively influences hippocampal neurogenesis (3).

Its mental health benefits do not only stem from physiologic mechanisms. From a psychological standpoint, exercise builds self-efficacy. Regardless of your level of fitness, there is always potential for personal growth, be it walking an extra five minutes, swimming an extra lap or lifting a few extra pounds. The process of setting and attaining goals can increase self-confidence.

In addition, exercise can protect you from burnout. A systematic review found that exercise is an effective intervention for reducing burnout among healthcare workers (4). Another study conducted at the Mayo Clinic found that resident and fellow physicians who participated in a team-based, incentivized exercise program reported higher quality of life and reduced burnout compared to nonparticipants (5). Furthermore, another systematic review consisting of 11,500 medical students across 13 countries found that physical activity was associated with reduced burnout and improved quality of life (6).

Considering its health benefits, it is unfortunate that exercise is often the first activity sacrificed from our packed schedules. On the surface, this decision is understandable because exercise requires time and energy, both of which are at a premium. However, being busy is not the only reason physicians ditch exercise. Being perfectionists with an all-or-nothing mentality makes it harder to stick to an exercise routine.

As an example, I worked with a physician who had completely stopped exercising during her residency training. She used to be an avid runner and had completed a number of half-marathons. She was frustrated that she had lost muscle mass and gained weight during residency.

During an afternoon session, I asked her about her plans that evening, which included dinner with her husband. I noted a gap in her schedule and wondered how she would feel if she went for a light jog. She was initially reluctant because she was not as fit as she used to be. She dreaded facing the decline in her physical conditioning. However, she also recalled feeling better about herself when she used to exercise. She acknowledged that a light jog would do wonders for her mood even if it was not the same intensity or duration as past workouts. She agreed to be kind to herself and focus on the present moment rather than make comparisons to a previous version of herself. This conversation was the catalyst that helped her reintegrate exercise in her schedule.

As achievement-oriented perfectionists, we set the bar high in every facet of our lives including our workouts. We expect a workout to last a good hour and include a predetermined set of vigorous exercises. In our minds, if a workout does not meet these criteria, then it does not count and is not worth our time.

The reality is that some exercise is better than no exercise. Even a 20-minute brisk walk or 15-minute stretch is better than no physical activity. Sure, the American Heart Association recommends 150 minutes of moderate-intensity aerobic activity per week. However, you would never tell a patient not to exercise just because they could not meet this guideline. Letting go of perfectionistic ideals creates time and space for exercise to be an integral part of your lifestyle.

When incorporating physical activity, focus primarily on building the habit of exercising consistently. If exercise becomes an integral part of your identity, you will automatically find time for it. Be patient with yourself as it can take months to build a new habit (7). Adjusting the intensity and duration of your workouts to meet personal fitness goals falls secondary to the primary goal of solidifying the habit of exercising consistently. Many people fail to stick to an exercise regimen because they try to achieve too much too fast, which sets them up for disappointment and injury.

Nutrition

Eating fruits and vegetables is no antidote for the systemic factors that have fragmented the healthcare system and tarnished the practice of medicine. However, there is evidence that healthy eating habits can play a protective role against burnout. A cross-sectional study of 630 employees in Finland showed that frequent consumption of healthy food items had an inverse relationship with burnout (8). Another cross-sectional, multinational study of 2,623 healthcare providers found a significant positive association between burnout and higher fast-food consumption (9).

Removing processed foods from your diet would be ideal considering their negative health effects and addicting nature (10). However, perfectionism is the enemy of progress. Instead of depriving yourself of such foods, focus first on incorporating healthy, nutritious options. If you have a sweet tooth, grab an apple or banana instead of a muffin. Choose yogurt over ice cream. Focus first on building the taste for healthy options. I have had patients tell me they found soda too sweet after consistently choosing water to quench their thirst or rice too bloating once they made the switch to chopped cauliflower. The key is to have healthy options to lean on. The more you can satisfy your appetite through healthy options, the less you need to rely on unhealthy ones.

Preparing in advance can help you make wiser choices. As a personal example, I pack my lunch for work the night before. This habit prevents me from making the trip to a local plaza during my lunch break that is only a three-minute drive from my office. It is a mecca of fast-food options that would leave me feeling bloated and lethargic for the afternoon clinic.

Am I perfect in enforcing this habit? No. Have I occasionally skipped my packed lunch for a quick, greasy burger even though I know I will ultimately regret it? You bet. The goal is not to be perfect, but to make healthy choices the majority of time.

Avoid Alcohol

The negative health effects of alcohol are well documented (11). Unfortunately, physicians are not immune to this vice. A systematic review involving 51,680 physicians from 17 countries found an increase in problematic alcohol use from 16.3% to 26.8% over a 15-year span (12).

A survey of U.S. physicians found 12.9% of male physicians and 21.4% of female physicians met diagnostic criteria for alcohol abuse or dependence (13). Of note, the survey had a response rate of only 26.7%. Let's be real. How many physicians do you think skipped the survey because they were too afraid to admit their own problematic pattern of drinking? I would not be surprised if the number of physicians meeting diagnostic criteria for alcohol use disorder was even higher.

If you consistently have a drink or two at the end of the workday to unwind and forget about the day's stressors, you are playing with fire. The danger is even greater if you drink alone. Using alcohol as a reward comes with risk. Over time, you can develop tolerance to its anxiolytic effects and require greater quantities to get the same effect. This is how alcohol gets you entangled in its web, one innocent drink at a time.

The need to unwind is completely understandable considering the stressful nature of our profession. However, relying on healthier alternatives is essential. Meditation, journaling, deep breathing exercises and muscle relaxation techniques can effectively calm your body and mind without any associated risks.

Connection

The relationship between loneliness and burnout is bidirectional. Not only does burnout have a negative effect on your relationship with loved ones, but feeling lonely makes you prone to burnout. A cross-sectional study of 486 participants found that loneliness is a risk factor for burnout (14).

Loneliness remains quite prevalent despite technological advances intended to improve social connectedness by overcoming time and geographic barriers. According to a national survey of nearly 2,500 U.S. adults, 58% of participants reported feeling lonely consistently (15). Loneliness comes at a great risk not only to your mental health, but also your physical health. A meta-analysis linked loneliness to a 29% increased risk of developing coronary heart disease and a 32% increased risk of stroke (16). A prospective cohort study of 580,182 individuals found that social isolation increases the risk of premature death (17). According to experts, loneliness carries a mortality risk that is comparable to smoking 15 cigarettes per day and even exceeds the health risks of obesity (18).

In an attempt to overcome loneliness, people often focus on increasing the quantity of their relationships. A reasonable strategy is to pursue personal interests with the goal of meeting other people who share them. As a personal example, I play basketball at the local rec center on Thursday mornings with other men. When we are not competing on the court, we often talk about our personal lives. Though brief, these conversations are meaningful and add a layer of connection to my life.

However, it is equally important to strengthen the quality of your current relationships. A study of 2,723 couples found that frequent negative interactions between spouses can enhance feelings of loneliness (19).

On a daily basis, I work with patients who feel profoundly lonely in their marriage or partnership.

Increasing the number of your relationships is not a substitute for improving the quality of your existing ones. Relationships are hard work. The odds are stacked against you when it comes to being at the right place and time to meet the right person and grow with them together for the rest of your life. You need to be intentional if you want your closest relationships to be more fulfilling. Here are three tips to help you.

First of all, there will be times that you feel upset with your partner. Press pause before reflexively unleashing your thoughts and feelings. It is better to stay silent for a few seconds rather than say or do something you will regret years down the road.

However, you can bite your tongue for only so long. It is important to express your thoughts and feelings in an effective manner. Though important, we do not know how to express ourselves. In her book titled "The Relationship Skills Workbook," Dr. Julia B Colwell presents the S.E.W. technique for expressing yourself. The S stands for expressing your body sensations. Examples can include tension around your jaw, neck and shoulders, heaviness in your chest or knots in your stomach. The E stands for expressing the emotion associated with the body sensations. For example, stomach knots may indicate you are scared or heaviness in your chest that you are sad. Finally, the W stands for expressing your wants and needs (20).

Let's assume you are frustrated with your spouse because they don't take their dirty plates to the sink after dinner. The sight of the dishes on the table triggers body sensations and associated emotions. Observe them and find the words to express them before making a request. You may say something like:

> I feel chest and neck tightness every time I see dirty dishes on the table. I think I feel disregarded and sad when this happens. It would mean a lot to me if you took your plates to the sink after dinner.

This approach reduces the odds of conflict escalation. You are not blaming your partner or making accusatory statements. You are taking ownership of your physical and emotional experience. Sharing your experience with your partner helps them better understand on a deeper level the impact of their behavior which can motivate them to change.

This leads to the final tip which is to have empathy for them. Emotionally understanding your loved ones is psychological oxygen for them. When a loved one presents with a problem, the reflex is to try and fix it. Though reasonable, this is not the best approach. By immediately jumping into problem-solving mode, you may inadvertently convey the following message: "Let's solve your problem as fast as we can so we can move on because I don't want to deal with this any longer than I have to."

Another downside of prematurely jumping into problem-solving mode is not collecting all pertinent data to offer personalized advice. You may cut them short and prevent them from fully sharing what is transpiring. As a result, you may offer cookie-cutter advice which is not as effective.

A healthier approach is to express empathy for what your partner is going through. Validate their emotional experience. Give them the safe space to express themselves. Listen intently. Seek to understand with genuine interest and curiosity. You do not need to solve their stressor. Feeling seen, heard and understood is the catalyst that will help them overcome it. Having space to process what is transpiring can lead to new insights which will help them come up with their own solutions.

Spirituality

In general, the literature is fairly limited about the association between spirituality and physician burnout. This is unfortunate because spirituality can be a valuable source of meaning, support and inspiration in one's life. Believing in something bigger than you can protect you from the existential crisis of struggling to make sense of our finite time on this earth.

There is evidence that spirituality can protect physicians from burnout. A study found that resident physicians who engaged in an active spiritual life were less susceptible to burnout (21). Another study of medical and mental health professionals attending palliative care seminars found that daily spiritual experiences can lessen occupational burnout (22).

Failing to acknowledge the central role that spirituality plays for many of our colleagues carries the risk of marginalizing them. A meta-analysis of 3,342 physicians from seven countries showed the majority of respondents had a religious affiliation, with half of the participants reporting their religious beliefs influenced how they practiced medicine (23).

It is important that medical training and healthcare institutions carve out the necessary time and space for clinicians to practice their spiritual beliefs. It is equally important that clinicians explore their own personal beliefs. They can be a vital source of meaning and purpose in life.

Sleep

Sleep disturbances are common among physicians. This should not be surprising when you consider our work schedule includes long hours, night shifts and weekends. A cross-sectional study of over 1,000 faculty and staff members in a teaching hospital found that 29% met criteria for at least one sleeping disorder, with over 90% of cases being undiagnosed and untreated. It also showed that screening positive for a sleep disorder was associated with burnout and reduced professional fulfillment (24).

Prioritizing your sleep is essential for your physical and mental health. Engaging in healthy sleep hygiene can help with sleep onset and maintenance. Do your best to go to bed at a reasonable time. Be mindful of your caffeine consumption. With a half-life of about five hours, a cup of coffee in the afternoon can interfere with sleep onset. Avoid alcohol, heavy meals and consuming liquids at night. Do not use electronics while in bed. Engage in a calming routine to prepare yourself for bedtime such as having a warm shower, doing some light stretching or a brief meditation.

Rest

Rest can take on a variety of different forms. You can rest while reading a book, laying on your lawn, doing a puzzle, stretching your body or spending time with a loved one. Finding time to recharge your batteries is challenging due to working long hours. Adding family and social responsibilities to the mix only makes rest more elusive.

However, time constraints are not the only reason you barely rest. There are also emotional forces that prevent you from resting. The culture of medicine has trained you to put the needs of others ahead of your own. Prioritizing your needs can feel uncomfortable, even prohibitive, when you are surrounded by colleagues who work tirelessly from dawn to dusk or senior physicians who criticize the 80-hour weekly work limit for physicians-in-training, established by the ACGME, because they used to work longer hours during their training.

Sacrificing self-care feels like the path of least resistance in such an intense, hypercompetitive environment. You don't want to stand apart as not having the same level of dedication as your peers. However, sacrificing self-care comes with great consequences. From a practical standpoint, not getting adequate rest makes it exponentially harder to keep up with the demands of your busy life. It can be difficult to muster the necessary energy, concentration and stamina to make it through a demanding day when you have not taken the necessary time to recharge your batteries. This also makes you more vulnerable to making mistakes at work which could compromise patient care.

From a psychological standpoint, sacrificing self-care negatively impacts your relationship with yourself. Constantly prioritizing everyone's wants and needs ahead of your own implies that your needs, and subsequently you, are not as important.

Imagine if your loved ones followed in your footsteps and operated the same way. How would you feel if you witnessed them jeopardize their physical and mental health to fulfill professional responsibilities? Would you encourage them to make such a sacrifice?

The answer is a resounding No. You would certainly encourage them to prioritize their needs even if it meant changing jobs. No job is worth sacrificing one's health. Yet, as physicians, we often don't heed our own advice as we work ourselves to the point of exhaustion and depletion.

Actions speak louder than words. Your words will fall on deaf ears if you don't practice what you preach. If you encourage loved ones to prioritize their self-care, but never take a break yourself, then you are creating a double standard which lessens your credibility. I have worked with countless patients who struggled taking a break because their parents were always on the go. They beat themselves up for not being able to maintain the same ferocious pace as their parents, even if they had been reassured by them that it's ok to take a break.

Being constantly busy is not the equivalent of being productive. It is often an avoidance behavior. Many people are always on the go in a desperate attempt to avoid difficult thoughts, feelings or situations. For example, I have worked with patients who worked day and night to avoid addressing a failing marriage or troubles within a household. In some ways, being inundated with work is easier and more familiar than dealing with intimate problems behind closed doors. However, avoidance never works. Avoiding problems does not make them go away. It only provides the necessary time and space for them to grow into bigger problems.

Cognitive reframes can help you prioritize rest by conceptualizing it differently. First, look at self-care as a necessity rather than a luxury. Taking breaks is essential to be more efficient and effective in your daily life. You spend the majority of your day giving yourself to your family, friends and patients. Putting fuel in your tank is essential to keep on serving others.

In addition, self-care is not a selfish act. Making yourself a priority is not just about meeting your needs. It models this behavior for the people who matter most to you. Finding a way to integrate a dose of self-care in your busy schedule can show loved ones how to fulfill competing responsibilities without completely sacrificing their health and happiness in the process.

Finally, being surrounded by type A workaholics can make self-care seem like a sign of weakness. Remember that you are not a machine, but a human being who needs rest. The ability to go against the grain and advocate for yourself in such a hypercompetitive environment is a sign of strength and resilience, not weakness.

In summary, prioritizing your physical, mental and social health is essential to protect yourself from burnout. Healthy habits such as exercise, getting adequate sleep and spending quality time with loved ones do not address the systemic factors that contribute to your suffering. However, they mitigate their impact on you and help you be better equipped to navigate work stressors. Compromising your health only makes this process exponentially harder.

References

1. Kane L. 'I cry but no one cares': physician burnout and depression report 2023. *Medscape*. January 27, 2023. Accessed October 14, 2023. https://www.medscape.com/slideshow/2023-lifestyle-burnout-6016058
2. Medisauskaite A, Kamau C. Does occupational distress raise the risk of alcohol use, binge-eating, ill health and sleep problems among medical doctors? A UK cross-sectional study. *BMJ Open*. 2019 May 15;9(5):e027362. doi:10.1136/bmjopen-2018-027362
3. Anderson E, Shivakumar G. Effects of exercise and physical activity on anxiety. *Front Psychiatry*. 2013 Apr 23;4:27. doi:10.3389/fpsyt.2013.00027
4. Naczenski LM, Vries JD, Hooff MLMV, Kompier MAJ. Systematic review of the association between physical activity and burnout. *J Occup Health*. 2017;59(6):477–494. doi:10.1539/joh.17-0050-RA
5. Seward MW, Marso CC, Soled DR, Briggs LG. Medicine in motion: addressing physician burnout through fitness, philanthropy, and interdisciplinary community building. *Am J Lifestyle Med*. 2020 Dec 29;16(4):462–468. doi:10.1177/1559827620983782
6. Taylor CE, Scott EJ, Owen K. Physical activity, burnout and quality of life in medical students: a systematic review. *Clin Teach*. 2022;19(6):e13525. doi:10.1111/tct.13525
7. Lally P, van Jaarsveld CHM, Potts HWW, Wardle J. How are habits formed: modelling habit formation in the real world. *European Journal of Social Psychology*. 2010;40(6):998–1009. https://doi.org/10.1002/ejsp.674
8. Penttinen MA, Virtanen J, Laaksonen M, et al. The association between healthy diet and burnout symptoms among Finnish municipal employees. *Nutrients*. 2021 Jul 13;13(7):2393. doi:10.3390/nu13072393
9. Alexandrova-Karamanova A, Todorova I, Montgomery A, et al. Burnout and health behaviors in health professionals from seven European countries. *Int Arch Occup Environ Health*. 2016;89:1059–1075. doi:10.1007/s00420-016-1143-5
10. Lustig RH. Ultraprocessed food: addictive, toxic, and ready for regulation. *Nutrients*. 2020 Nov 5;12(11):3401. doi:10.3390/nu12113401
11. Varghese J, Dakhode S. Effects of alcohol consumption on various systems of the human body: a systematic review. *Cureus*. 2022 Oct 8;14(10):e30057. doi:10.7759/cureus.30057
12. Wilson J, Tanuseputro P, Myran DT, et al. Characterization of problematic alcohol use among physicians: a systematic review. *JAMA Netw Open*. 2022 Dec 1;5(12):e2244679. doi:10.1001/jamanetworkopen.2022.44679

13. Oreskovich MR, Shanafelt T, Dyrbye LN, et al. The prevalence of substance use disorders in American physicians. *The American Journal of Addictions.* 2015;24(1):30–38. https://doi.org/10.1111/ajad.12173

14. Card KG, Bodner A, Li R, et al. Loneliness and social support as key contributors to burnout among Canadians workers in the third wave of the COVID-19 pandemic: a cross-sectional study. *J Occup Health.* 2022;64(1):e12360. doi:10.1002/1348-9585.12360

15. The Cigna Group. The loneliness epidemic persists: a post-pandemic look at the state of loneliness among U.S. adults. 2021. https://newsroom.thecignagroup.com/loneliness-epidemic-persists-post-pandemic-look

16. Valtorta NK, Kanaan M, Gilbody S, et al. Loneliness and social isolation as risk factors for coronary heart disease and stroke: systematic review and meta-analysis of longitudinal observational studies. *Heart* 2016;102:1009–1016. https://doi.org/10.1136/heartjnl-2015-308790

17. Alcaraz KI, Eddens KS, Blase JL, et al. Social isolation and mortality in US black and white men and women. *American Journal of Epidemiology.* 2019;188(1):102–109. https://doi.org/10.1093/aje/kwy231

18. Sweet J. The loneliness pandemic. The psychology and social costs of isolation in everyday life. *The Harvard Magazine.* January-February 2021. https://www.harvardmagazine.com/2020/12/feature-the-loneliness-pandemic

19. Ayalon L, Shiovitz-Ezra S, Palgi Y. Associations of loneliness in older married men and women. *Aging & Mental Health.* 2013;17(1):33–39. doi:10.1080/13607863.2012.702725

20. Colwell J. The relationship skills workbook: a do-it-yourself guide to a thriving relationship. *Sounds True.* October, 2014.

21. Doolittle BR, Windish DM, Seelig CB. Burnout, coping, and spirituality among internal medicine resident physicians. *J Grad Med Educ.* 2013;5:257–261. doi:10.4300/JGME-D-12-00136.1.

22. Holland JM, Neimeyer RA. Reducing the risk of burnout in end-of-life care settings: the role of daily spiritual experiences and training. *Palliative and Supportive Care.* 2005;3(3):173–181. doi:10.1017/S1478951505050297

23. Kørup AK, Søndergaard J, Lucchetti G, et al. Religious values of physicians affect their clinical practice: a meta-analysis of individual participant data from 7 countries. *Medicine (Baltimore).* 2019;98(38):e17265. doi:10.1097/MD.0000000000017265

24. Weaver MD, Robbins R, Quan SF, et al. Association of sleep disorders with physician burnout. *JAMA Netw Open.* 2020 Oct 1;3(10):e2023256. doi:10.1001/jamanetworkopen.2020.23256

8 Let Go of Imposter Syndrome

In our fiercely competitive society, achievement has become a top priority. This is especially true in medicine where type A perfectionists make tremendous sacrifices over a long period of time to achieve their professional goals.

It is completely understandable to feel proud of yourself for becoming a physician. Many have aspired to be in your position, but failed to achieve this goal. It took a great deal of grit, persistence and resilience to make it through medical school, let alone residency and fellowship training. The same holds true for being an attending physician. Showing up to serve on the frontline of human suffering takes great perseverance.

Unfortunately, I have worked with countless physicians who have lost sight of the magnitude of their achievement. They suffer from imposter syndrome which is the persistent belief that their success is the result of mere luck rather than personal ability, skill and effort. They fear their abilities have been overrated all along and that others will eventually discover the truth about them.

Imposter syndrome is not merely the experience of self-doubt, which is a healthy response to new situations. Being 100% sure of yourself at all times is a sign of both arrogance and ignorance. Such an approach makes you vulnerable to careless mistakes stemming from blind spots. It is appropriate to momentarily question yourself when facing unique clinical situations or transitioning to a new role with increased responsibilities.

In contrast, imposter syndrome is characterized by a repeated questioning of one's abilities. There is a persistent fear of being exposed as incompetent.

Imposter syndrome is common among physicians. A national survey of 3,237 U.S. physicians showed that 59.6% of participants scored in the moderate, frequent or intense range on the Clance Imposter Phenomenon Scale. The same survey also showed that imposter syndrome was a risk factor for burnout. In particular, there was an increase in emotional

DOI: 10.4324/9781003473923-12

exhaustion and depersonalization along with a decrease in personal fulfillment among individuals with higher degrees of imposter syndrome (1).

The high prevalence of imposter syndrome may seem like a paradox when you consider the amount of skill, ability and resilience it takes to ultimately become a physician. What are the odds that you became a physician by mere luck when you consider the number of attending physicians who supervised you during your medical training and the gauntlet of examinations you had to pass? You deserve to be a physician and worked hard to earn the privilege of serving in this role.

Feeling like an imposter may not be based on objective data, but can have a profound impact. One of its manifestations is when physicians perpetually extend their training in a desperate attempt to avoid becoming attendings because of not feeling prepared. As an example, I worked with a physician about to complete his fellowship training. He was having tremendous anxiety about his upcoming graduation. Experiencing some anxiety during a career transition is understandable. When you are a physician-in-training, there is comfort in having an attending supervise your work and sign off on your clinical notes. It can take some time getting used to no longer having this safety net.

However, his anxiety was disproportionate to the situation at hand. He felt no joy for finally completing the odyssey of becoming a physician. He was reluctant to let go of the role of being a student as he dreaded the upcoming transition. His fears were not warranted as he had passed all required standardized exams and received glowing performance reviews from supervising physicians during his training.

One of the goals of our work together was to reduce his anxiety by identifying and challenging the factors that were fueling his imposter syndrome.

Let's explore some of these factors and how you can overcome them.

Social Comparisons

Social comparison theory was first popularized by psychologist Leon Festinger in 1954. It theorized that we use others as a measuring stick to evaluate our own abilities and skills (2).

You have compared yourself to peers from a young age. As a high school and college student, you stood apart from the crowd by earning strong grades and participating in extracurricular activities. Odds are you would have not made it into medical school if you were an average college student with a lackluster resume. Keeping track of your performance against peers was essential to getting into medical school.

Social comparisons only continued during medical school. Your class ranking influenced whether you would be accepted into your specialty of choice or train in a desirable region. For more competitive specialties, being an average medical student would not suffice.

Measuring your performance against peers helped you succeed in your professional life. At the same time, this tendency is a double-edged sword that has made you vulnerable to imposter syndrome and burnout (3). Being immersed in a work environment with colleagues who are achievement-oriented, hardworking perfectionists and constantly comparing yourself to them can make you lose sight of how much you have accomplished. The shine from your personal achievements has faded away because you compare yourself to other physicians who have also overcome similar trials and tribulations.

Though prevalent, social comparisons often entail distorted thought patterns which cloud your perspective. Understanding them is important to avoid the negative effects from comparing yourself to others.

First of all, studies show we generally compare ourselves to those who seem superior in some way, even if such comparisons pose a threat to our self-esteem and mood (4). Feelings of inadequacy can bubble to the surface when you only fixate on physicians who appear to be more competent or successful than you. It is easy to look ahead and forget the mass of people who aspired to be in your shoes but failed to enter the pearly gates of medicine.

In addition, vertical comparisons are flawed because their focus is too narrow. They myopically focus on the parts of your life in which you feel behind. Yet, they ignore other areas in which you are ahead. As a result, they do not provide a complete picture of your standing in comparison to others.

To highlight this point, let me share a clinical example that does not involve a physician. I worked with an individual who felt ashamed to be raising his family in an apartment. He worked a blue-collar job and lacked the financial means to be a homeowner. He felt tremendous envy and shame every time his kids were invited by friends to their homes because it was a painful reminder that he was not a homeowner.

During our work together, I asked him to take a complete inventory of his life. Despite living in close quarters, he was happily married. He enjoyed a strong bond with his children who were thriving socially and academically. His loved ones were healthy and happy. Did he ever consider the possibility that many in his social circle, who owned homes, did not enjoy the same blessings? Perhaps they were going through difficulties he was unaware of such as marital conflict or health problems. Maybe they had overextended themselves financially and were struggling to keep up with the monthly mortgage payment. Adopting a more complete picture helped him realize that even though he felt behind in one aspect of life, he was ahead in others.

You might be in a similar situation. You might not have your dream job, but a family you are proud of. You might be single but surrounded by people who love you. Money might be tight because you are drowning in student loans but your life may be rich in experiences. Keeping the whole picture in mind can protect you from the distortions hidden within social comparisons.

Furthermore, social comparisons are often based on appearances. You compare your real, messy life against someone who *appears* to have more of what you want. For example, when someone drives by in a luxury car, you may assume they are in a better financial position. However, how can you be certain this is the case? What if they took out significant debt to lease the car and are struggling to make the monthly payment?

Your physician colleagues are no different. They project a façade of how they want to be perceived. They hide their worries, struggles and insecurities behind a façade of degrees, titles and white coats. Realizing that social comparisons are often based on appearances can reduce their negative impact on you.

Finally, remember that social comparisons are a moving target. After achieving any goal, it is only a matter of time before you start comparing yourself to a new set of people who appear further ahead than you. When you were a broke medical student, you compared yourself to other broke classmates. When you were a resident, you compared yourself to other residents. As an attending, the target has moved and you focus on other attendings or successful people in your social circle. The target never stops moving. Even billionaires compare themselves to other billionaires. In the words of Gary Shteyngart, who interviewed billionaires for his novel Lake Success (5):

> Here were people who could purchase anything they could ever want and whose wealth was widely envied, and even they weren't content. At the end of the day, I was just happy to end this research, because it was quite depressing.

Instead of relying on others, a more useful measuring stick is to focus on your personal journey. Keep track of where you have been, where you are and where you are heading. After all, success is not a zero-sum game because everyone is climbing a different mountain. Someone making it to the top of their mountain has no impact on whether you reach the top of your mountain.

However, if you need to compare yourself to your peers, substitute envy with curiosity. The success of others leaves behind clues that can help you achieve your personal goals. Studying their success with curiosity can be a great benefit to you.

Perfectionism

An additional factor that can contribute to imposter syndrome is perfectionism. Despite its role in medicine, perfectionistic traits are evident in those who struggle with imposter syndrome. A study found that students with imposter syndrome reported a greater concern over making mistakes, a tendency to overestimate the number of mistakes made, less confidence in their performance and greater anxiety both prior to and following tasks (6).

In many settings, the pursuit of perfection is necessary. I want my pilot to be perfect when flying a plane. The same holds true for a surgeon who is operating on a loved one or when a physician prescribes a medication. There is no margin for error in these scenarios. Any deviation in precision and accuracy can have devastating outcomes.

However, do you have to be perfect in every aspect of your life? I have worked with physicians whose perfectionism had spilled into their personal lives. They expected to keep their homes perfectly tidy even though they were raising young children who explore their environment by making messes. They also insisted on keeping their lawn perfectly manicured despite not having the free time to keep up with it. Their need for perfection was stifling their relationship with loved ones. In their desperate pursuit of perfection, they constantly jumped around different tasks without spending time with the people who mattered most.

Perfectionism can have a negative impact on your closest relationships. A study found that perfectionists experience significantly greater fear of intimacy (7). It is as if they are constantly on the go to avoid the vulnerability of intimacy. Their need to be perfect is a shield that hides perceived flaws and insecurities they are ashamed of.

Addressing perfectionism is essential when you consider its negative effects. This starts by remembering to be fair to yourself and others. You cannot be perfect in every aspect of your life. Something has to give as competing roles and responsibilities pull you in different directions. Be wise in how you allocate your time and energy.

As an example, I worked with a physician who would become upset every time he arrived home at the end of the workday to find a mess. The sight of an untidy house was so distressing that he would immediately start cleaning rather than interact with his spouse and young children who had not seen him all day.

During our work together, I asked him to consider the message he was sending his loved ones. His actions were telling his family that maintaining a tidy house was more important than spending quality time with them. Were his actions aligned with his values? If his family was the priority, could the cleaning routine not wait until after he had spent some quality time with them?

I also asked him to reflect on whether he was being fair to his spouse by expecting her to maintain a clean house. Raising young children is hard work. They do not sit still because their overactive minds learn by exploring their surrounding environment. His insistence on keeping the house tidy was interfering with this important developmental process. A healthier approach would be to let his children make a mess and then clean it together as a family. This would teach his children the valuable lesson of cleaning up after themselves. Instead, by cleaning up their mess on his own, he was teaching his children not to be accountable for their actions because someone else would magically take care of their mess.

Letting go of unrealistic expectations is essential to combat imposter syndrome. You cannot be perfect in every aspect of your life. If your work and family are your main priorities, then accept that other parts of your life, such as keeping up with social obligations, maintaining a manicured lawn or staying in tip top physical shape will fall through the cracks and that's ok. Every Yes comes with a No. Prioritizing one thing means you have to let go of something else. The best you can do is be intentional when making a trade-off.

At the same time, it is important to have realistic expectations of others. They cannot be perfect in every aspect of life either. They are human beings with flaws and imperfections like you and me. They excel in some parts of life and lag in others. Be fair by realizing that they are forced to make similar trade-offs. Letting go of your perfectionistic standards will lead to deeper, more authentic relationships.

Narcissism

An additional factor that can predispose you to imposter syndrome is narcissism. Including a section on this factor may seem surprising as narcissism appears to be less common among physicians compared to the general population (8). Nonetheless, we are all familiar with physicians whose strong narcissistic traits had a negative impact on team dynamics.

When you think of narcissism, the image that likely comes to mind is of the grandiose narcissist who is boastful and arrogant. You can recognize them from a mile away because they demand the spotlight. They brag about their achievements and can be forceful to get their way. They are not shy about using others to advance personal agendas. In general, they lack empathy and have little concern about how their actions negatively affect others.

However, there is a less known form of narcissism known as the vulnerable type. Such narcissists tend to hide from the spotlight even though they yearn for it. Despite being discreet, they harbor grandiose fantasies of validation. They are characterized by a fragile self-esteem, hypersensitivity to criticism and constant feelings of shame. They avoid feedback and may respond to constructive criticism with disproportionate anger.

Vulnerable narcissism is associated with higher levels of imposter syndrome. It is also negatively associated with different measures of well-being such as life satisfaction, autonomy, personal growth and self-acceptance (9). Since medicine exposes physicians to clinical encounters that are often high-stakes with uncertain outcomes, it is important for physicians to identify and address any underlying narcissistic traits that can impact their clinical performance and interactions with team members.

The Healthcare System

Finally, the healthcare system contributes to your imposter syndrome by placing unrealistic expectations on you. In response to financial difficulties, hospitals often ask physicians to work harder by squeezing more patients in their packed schedules and increasing annual work productivity benchmarks.

At the same time, hospitals often implement policies that are in conflict with each other. As an example, hospitals ask patients about their wait times on satisfaction surveys. It is reasonable for patients to expect to be seen in a timely manner because their time is valuable. The problem occurs when hospitals place too many patients on a physician's schedule which causes them to fall behind due to time constraints. This results in longer wait times for patients and lower satisfaction scores. In a desperate effort to avoid being late, a physician may rush through their patient encounters which also leaves patients dissatisfied. Ironically, scores on patient satisfaction surveys are often tied to physician pay, which highlights how physicians literally end up paying the price for being put in no-win situations.

It is completely understandable for hospitals to implement metrics that measure the quality of care delivered by physicians. The problem arises when hospitals put physicians in no-win situations. Such unfair demands are key drivers to imposter syndrome and burnout because they make physicians feel incompetent for failing to meet assigned targets. As physicians, it is in our nature to blame ourselves for shortcomings even if they are due to systemic factors.

A combination of systemic factors and individual traits explains why the majority of physicians suffer from imposter syndrome. Cultivating the virtue of humility can serve as a powerful antidote to reverse this trend.

Humility

Humility has a negative connotation because it is often confused with being weak, fragile and meek. Many consider humility as synonymous with being passive and letting others walk all over you. From this perspective, it stands in opposition to the Western ideal of staunch individualism where your dreams can become a reality as long as you work hard enough.

This is an inaccurate viewpoint. A more appropriate definition of humility is the ability to engage in an accurate assessment of one's characteristics by acknowledging strengths and limitations (10). When viewed from this prism, humility provides a powerful antidote to imposter syndrome, which stems from a hypercritical self-assessment that is clouded by unfair social comparisons and perfectionistic expectations (11).

Humble individuals are far from weak or fragile. It takes a great deal of strength and courage to engage in honest and accurate self-reflection. One has to be secure in themselves to conceptualize weaknesses as opportunities for self-improvement rather than blemishes to be ashamed of.

The truth is you are no better or worse than anyone else. You are a mere human, one of over 100 billion who have ever lived on earth (12). Regardless of how much status, power or money you have, the same inevitable fate awaits you as everyone else. You will die and be forgotten. It may be within the span of one generation or ten generations, but the ripple effect of your life will ultimately come to an end and no one will know that you ever existed.

Though initially anxiety-provoking, recognizing your inevitable fate is liberating. Understanding how small each one of us truly is in the grand scheme frees you from the shackles of social comparisons, perfectionistic tendencies and narcissistic façades. To think that you are better or worse than anyone is meaningless. This change in perspective allows you to embrace a more authentic life that is rooted in deeper, more meaningful values such as kindness, empathy and service. These values exemplify the idea that every life is inherently worthy regardless of one's gender, race, ethnicity, religious background or socioeconomic standing.

At the heart of humility is the ability to detach your self-worth from external measures of success. It is the recognition that your self-worth is not derived from titles, degrees, professional standing, accumulated wealth, material possessions, number of followers on social media or any other status symbol. Your self-worth is an essential, inherent and undeniable part of your humanity.

You are worthy because you are human. Period.

As a personal example, my father is a cook and my mother a cashier at a grocery store. Money was tight growing up but I am privileged to have grown up in a safe and loving home environment. With their love and support I became a physician which affords me a different lifestyle than what my parents could provide. Does becoming a physician make me a more worthy human being compared to my parents? The answer is a resounding No! This is because every human being is inherently worthy regardless of external measures of personal success. Being a physician does not make you more worthy than anyone else.

Cultivating the virtue of humility will help you let go of vertical social comparisons and stop overidealizing pursuits in a futile attempt to bolster your self-worth. Whether you are ahead in some parts of life and behind in others has no bearing on your self-worth.

Every single one of us is a mosaic of strengths and weaknesses. Some of the pieces of your mosaic are gold and diamonds. They represent your strengths, abilities and skills. Other pieces are coal which represents your weaknesses and flaws. Regardless of composition, every mosaic is unique and complete. This includes your mosaic.

The problem occurs when you fixate on only a few parts of your mosaic rather than its entirety. Focusing only on your positive attributes predisposes you to grandiosity and narcissism. Such a perspective comes with great risk. Your weaknesses and limitations are areas for improvement that need to be addressed. Ignoring these blind spots can make you vulnerable to critical mistakes.

At the same time, focusing exclusively on your shortcomings is a recipe for feeling inferior and inadequate. How can you not feel like an imposter when you magnify your weaknesses and neglect your strengths? This creates the illusion that you do not belong in medicine because all your peers appear to be more skilled and capable than you.

The benefit of humility is that it allows you to see your mosaic in its entirety. This protects you from oscillating between the extremes of shame and grandiosity, which are two sides of the same coin. You are whole and complete even though you have areas for improvement like everyone else.

Reflecting on our journeys to become physicians can be a source of humility. As a psychiatrist, my training after college consists of four years of medical school followed by four years of residency training. I have devoted a large portion of my life to study psychiatry, which is only a small sliver of medicine. However, there is so much information within psychiatry that escapes me. For example, I do not have the necessary qualifications to treat children. Nor do I have the necessary training to be a forensic psychiatrist or perform procedures such as electroconvulsive therapy.

However, let's assume I had hypothetically mastered every aspect of psychiatry by becoming board certified in all psychiatric subspecialties. Even in such an extreme case, there would be limits in my knowledge because the field of psychiatry has limitations. For example, our medication interventions are not effective for all patients and we need to better understand why some people respond favorably to standard treatments, while others do not. They also come with potential side effects. As the field of psychiatry continues to evolve, my hope is that more effective treatment modalities will emerge.

The same holds true for you. If you are a specialist, you have mastered a small sliver of medicine that is constantly evolving. If you are a generalist, you have a broad knowledge base but not necessarily at the same depth as a specialist with fellowship training. Regardless of your clinical background, there are limits in your knowledge and ability to treat another human being's physical and mental health conditions. The recognition of these limitations, despite the many years you sacrificed to become a physician, can be a valuable source of humility.

On an individual level, humility has a positive effect on self-awareness. It invites you to engage in honest self-reflection that is not obscured by the toxic effects of shame or grandiosity. Recognizing that you are prone to blind spots spares you from the trap of overconfidence which jeopardizes clinical judgment and decision-making. Humble people tend to make more thorough, well-informed decisions (13).

Humility also has a positive effect on an interpersonal level. Humble individuals are more open to receiving feedback and considering opposing viewpoints. They are more willing to explore and learn from different perspectives. This promotes social cohesion and reconciliation. Considering the different types of bias that plague medicine, cultivating humility in healthcare systems can promote self-reflection, mitigate power imbalances and enhance institutional accountability (14).

Humility gives you the courage to say "I don't know" when you do not have the answer to your patient's or colleague's question. You appear more relatable and trustworthy by being honest rather than giving a circumstantial, round-about answer in a desperate attempt to hide your lack of knowledge. Saying "I don't know" does not mean that you are throwing in the towel and abandoning your patient. It is the recognition that you have reached the limits of your knowledge and have more to learn.

There are also times when we exhaust conventional treatment options. Even in this scenario, you can find creative and meaningful ways to be of service that extend beyond the traditional medical model. As an example, there have been times when I have exhausted all pharmacological options to treat a patient's treatment resistant depression. Even in this scenario, there were alternative ways to be helpful such as complete paperwork that helped the patient keep their job during their bout of depression, explore ways to increase their social support or write a letter for an emotional support animal that provided them comfort during their ordeal.

Limitations do not make you an imposter. They are inherent in medicine. There are limited treatment options for a host of medical conditions such as neurodegenerative disorders or different types of cancer. Recognizing that you have reached the limits of your knowledge and treatment options forces you to think outside the box and explore alternative ways to be helpful. Though overlooked, psychosocial interventions can have a profound impact on our patients.

Beware of the physician who does not recognize their limits! Their lack of self-awareness makes them vulnerable to blind spots and biases. Having the humility to acknowledge your limits makes you a better physician.

References

1. Shanafelt TD, Dyrbye LN, Sinsky C, et al. Imposter phenomenon in US physicians relative to the US working population. *Mayo Clin Proc*. 2022;97(11):1981–1993. doi:10.1016/j.mayocp.2022.06.021
2. Festinger L. A theory of social comparison processes. *Human Relations*. 1954;7(2):117–140. https://doi.org/10.1177/001872675400700202
3. Buunk AP, Zurriaga R, Peíro JM. Social comparison as a predictor of changes in burnout among nurses. *Anxiety Stress Coping*. 2010;23(2):181–194. doi:10.1080/10615800902971521
4. Gerber JP, Wheeler L, Suls J. A social comparison theory meta-analysis 60+ years on. *Psychological Bulletin*. 2018;144(2):177–197. https://doi.org/10.1037/bul0000127
5. Pinsker, J. The reason many ultrarich people aren't satisfied with their wealth. *The Atlantic*. December 4, 2018. Accessed April 9, 2024. https://www.theatlantic.com/family/archive/2018/12/rich-people-happy-money/577231/
6. Thompson T, Foreman P, Martin F. Impostor fears and perfectionistic concern over mistakes. *Personality and Individual Differences*. Oct 2000;29(4):629–647. https://doi.org/10.1016/S0191-8869(99)00218-4
7. Martin JL, Ashby JS. Perfectionism and fear of intimacy: implications for relationships. *The Family Journal*. 2004;12(4):368–374. https://doi.org/10.1177/1066480704267279
8. Bucknall V, Burwaiss S, MacDonald D, Charles K, Clement R. Mirror mirror on the ward, who's the most narcissistic of them all? Pathologic personality traits in health care. *CMAJ*. 2015;187(18):1359–1363. doi:10.1503/cmaj.151135
9. Kaufman SB, Weiss B, Miller JD, Campbell WK. Clinical correlates of vulnerable and grandiose narcissism: a personality perspective. *J Pers Disord*. 2020;34(1):107–130. doi:10.1521/pedi_2018_32_384
10. Tangney JP. Humility: theoretical perspectives, empirical findings and directions for future research. *J Soc Clin Psychol*. 2000; 19(1):70–82. https://doi.org/10.1521/jscp.2000.19.1.70
11. Michalec B, Gómez-Morales A, Tilburt JC, Hafferty FW. Examining impostor phenomenon through the lens of humility: spotlighting conceptual (dis)connections. *Mayo Clin Proc*. 2023;98(6):905–914. doi:10.1016/j.mayocp.2023.01.020
12. Haub C, Kaneda T. How many people have ever lived on earth? *PRB*. Nov 15, 2022. Accessed July 11, 2024. https://www.prb.org/articles/how-many-people-have-ever-lived-on-earth/

13. Porter T, Elnakouri A, Meyers EA, Shibayama T, Jayawickreme E, Grossmann I. Predictors and consequences of intellectual humility. *Nat Rev Psychol.* 2022;1(9):524–536. doi:10.1038/s44159-022-00081-9
14. Elbanna MF, Thomas MR, Patel PR, McHenry MS. Cultivating cultural humility to address the healthcare burnout epidemic – why it matters. *Glob Adv Integr Med Health*. 2023;12:27536130231162350. Published 2023 May 11. doi:10.1177/27536130231162350

9 Guard the Gate

You return home from a busy work day. The weather is perfect. You grab your favorite beverage from the fridge and head outside to your backyard deck to enjoy the sights and sounds of a lovely summer evening.

However, there is something peculiar about this evening. You are greeted by your neighbor who is mowing your lawn. At first, you might be surprised by their act of generosity and kindness. You might wonder if they have an ulterior motive. You ultimately convince yourself they have good intentions and are relieved that you don't have to mow your lawn for the next few days.

After mowing your lawn, they head off only to return with a shovel. They start digging in your backyard because they want you to have a garden. They insist it would be good for you to grow your own vegetables. How would you feel in this scenario? Odds are your initial pleasant feelings would be replaced by frustration and irritability. You have likely had enough of your neighbor and are eager for them to leave your property.

Your emotional shift would be completely understandable because your neighbor has crossed a line. They do not have the autonomy or authority to dig holes in your backyard without asking first for your permission. There was never a conversation about whether you wanted a garden to begin with. Instead, they violated the physical boundary separating your property from theirs by imposing their values onto you.

Boundaries define areas of ownership and responsibility. This is apparent with physical boundaries which delineate two neighboring properties. You are responsible for maintaining your plot of land and could be penalized for relinquishing your responsibility. At the same time, you get to decide what to do with your plot of land. You get to pick whether you plant a garden in your backyard or not.

Similar to the physical boundaries delineating two neighboring properties, there are emotional and social boundaries between you and others. These boundaries are derived from your different roles, each of which comes with its own set of perks and expectations.

DOI: 10.4324/9781003473923-13

As an example, being a parent comes with its own set of responsibilities. You are expected to keep your children safe. This is harder than it sounds. It only takes a few seconds of distraction for a toddler to climb a chair to perform an acrobatic jump. You are also expected to provide your children with food, shelter and clothing. This can be a challenging task when the toddler has a temper tantrum over their food options or insists on wearing their favorite red shirt from the dirty laundry pile. You cannot assign these responsibilities to anyone else. Failure to meet your parental responsibilities comes with punishment such as being reported to the authorities or losing custody of your children. At the same time, being a parent comes with perks. You get to form a special bond with your children, make memories with them and experience a type of love that enriches your life.

Being a physician comes with its own set of expectations. You are responsible for conducting yourself in a professional manner when interacting with patients. You also need to maintain adequate knowledge and follow the standard of care to meet their healthcare needs. Practicing medicine requires you to maintain an active medical license and complete continuing educational requirements. Your clinical decisions are expected to be in the best interest of your patients while respecting their autonomy. Fulfilling these responsibilities grants you the privilege of practicing medicine.

You hold a number of roles each of which comes with its own set of perks and responsibilities. Being in a romantic relationship is an example of this. The same holds true for being someone's friend or family member. Perhaps, you are an active church member who is expected to tithe and volunteer. You might run a side gig to make extra income. These different roles reflect the diversity of your skills, interests and relationships. They enrich your life by exposing you to a wide range of experiences.

At the same time, they make you vulnerable to burnout because competing work, family and social roles are vying for your limited time, attention and energy simultaneously. For example, your kids have soccer practice on the same evening that your employer wants you to attend a work meeting. Or you have to complete clinical notes at the end of the day which takes you away from loved ones. Your hospital employer might double book your schedule by assigning two patients at the same time slot and you have to decide which patient to see first. Competing responsibilities create moral dilemmas in which you have to pick which to prioritize.

It is impossible to be in two places simultaneously. You cannot be at a work meeting and your child's soccer practice at the same time. Nor can you do two things simultaneously. You cannot have a deep, meaningful conversation with your partner while writing quality clinical notes. You have to pick which responsibility to focus on.

Setting healthy boundaries is an effective strategy to combat burnout (1). It helps you regain some control over your busy life by focusing on what matters most at a particular moment. Telling your practice manager that you will not attend the evening work meeting because your child has soccer practice is an example of setting healthy boundaries. You are putting your family above work. The same holds true when you decline to attend a weekend social event because you need to stay home to recharge your batteries. You are choosing your health over a social responsibility.

There are two ways to set boundaries. The first is to say No when someone asks something from you. The second approach is to ask for help by delegating responsibilities to others. Though it may sound simple, setting boundaries is difficult. This is because there are emotional forces that interfere with your ability to set them.

In an attempt to avoid dealing with these difficult emotions, you often double down on your familiar pattern of working harder to overcome boundary violations. You may sacrifice time with yourself and loved ones by reluctantly agreeing to attend evening work meetings or taking on an unlimited number of assigned patients. It can emotionally feel easier to acquiesce to your employer's demands rather than set boundaries with them. You figure that if you try hard enough you will eventually find a way to keep up with everything.

Working harder to keep up with increasing expectations is not the solution. Sacrificing yourself to satisfy the needs of others is not a viable long-term strategy. This only gets you stuck in a vicious cycle of learned behavior in which people expect more out of you. They automatically approach you whenever they have a problem because they have grown accustomed to you solving them. In other words, the more you give, the more others expect you to give.

As an example, when a hospital goes through financially challenging times, their reflex is to ask physicians to work harder to generate more revenue. In response, we work harder to meet rising demands. The outcome is that hospitals have grown accustomed to asking physicians to do more every time a financial need arises rather than explore more sustainable solutions such as cutting back on administrative costs and eliminating systemic inefficiencies that lead to financial waste.

Getting stuck in a vicious cycle of working harder to meet increasing expectations is a path to burnout. It is only a matter of time before you collapse because too many responsibilities have been placed on your shoulders. A healthier and more sustainable approach is to become effective in setting healthy boundaries by overcoming the emotional barriers that interfere with this process. Let's dive into these emotional barriers and discuss strategies to overcome them.

Guilt

Guilt is the feeling that you have done something wrong. It arises from the difference between your actions and what you expect of yourself. Though distressing, guilt serves an important function. It provides a moral compass which reinforces prosocial behavior. The absence of guilt is a well-known characteristic of psychopathy (2).

The problem occurs when your guilt is excessive in intensity and duration. This can interfere with your ability to set healthy boundaries. When someone makes a request, you reluctantly agree because you feel like you are doing something wrong by saying No. As a result, you take on additional responsibilities despite already being busy and overwhelmed.

When I notice patients struggling with guilt, I remind them that there is no FDA approved medication for this emotion. You need to learn how to identify and process it. There are only two ways to cope with guilt. You can keep on saying Yes to every request to avoid feeling guilty or lower your expectations to a more realistic level. The problem with always saying Yes is that your life will ultimately spiral out of control. As a result, you need to learn how to cope with the guilt from saying No.

As an example, I worked with a resident physician whose family dynamics were causing her tremendous distress and interfering with her functioning at work. She would feel guilty for days after interacting with her mother. The guilt stemmed from her mother complaining that she was not being attentive to her.

The physician dreaded talking to her mother who was trying to entangle her in a codependent relationship. The mother was consumed with somatic experiences. Any time she experienced a physical symptom, the mother would call her primary care physician or rush to the local Emergency Department. The mother had undergone every imaginable medical test to uncover the source of her vague physical symptoms. Yet, every test result came back normal.

The mother frequently asked the resident for medical advice on what was afflicting her. Efforts to reassure her mother based on objective medical data were interpreted as being uncaring. The mother was blind to the underlying emotional forces reinforcing her physical symptoms. Taking on the sick role allowed her to receive both attention and financial support from family members.

One of the primary goals of therapy was to help this physician overcome feelings of guilt that were preventing her from setting boundaries with her mother. She felt like a terrible daughter every time she attempted to distance herself from the situation.

To overcome guilt, I asked her to reflect on what being a good daughter looks like. Was entering a codependent relationship with her mother a prerequisite for fulfilling that role? Would she expect this from anyone else in a similar situation? Could she still be empathetic to her mother without completely sacrificing herself in the process? Did being a good daughter depend on earning her mother's approval? Reflecting on these questions helped the physician realize that being a good daughter did not depend on meeting her mother's unfair expectations. The best she could do was set healthy boundaries to avoid being tangled in a codependent relationship that would only drag her down with the rest of her family.

To better understand if feelings of guilt are warranted, it is important to examine whether you have set your bar of expectations at a realistic level. To do this, remove yourself from the situation and imagine a person you love is in it. They are facing a similar dilemma but are having a hard time saying No due to feelings of guilt. What advice would you give them? Would you tell them to give in to the demands of others or would you encourage them to stand up for themselves?

The advice you give a loved one is the blueprint for how to proceed in your own situation. If you would encourage someone else to say No, then why is it not ok for you to say No? In other words, why the double standard? This discrepancy is evidence that you are being overly hard on yourself because you expect more out of yourself than others.

Lowering your bar of expectations to a more sustainable level may initially feel uncomfortable because you are used to reflexively stepping up and finding a way to juggle one more responsibility. However, your approach is not sustainable in the long run. It is a recipe for eventually collapsing from the collective weight of competing responsibilities.

Shame

Shame is the feeling you are inherently flawed and not worthy of love. Unlike guilt, which refers to one's behavior, shame refers to one's being. It is the fear that people won't like you if they knew who you really are. To compensate, we put up our guard and hide the parts of ourselves we are ashamed of.

Shame interferes with boundary setting when you believe you are not worthy of advocating for yourself. If you consider yourself unworthy, then you won't view your needs as important. As a result, you are more likely to respond to boundary violations with silence rather than by standing up for yourself.

Staying silent may feel easier in the moment, but it comes at a cost. First of all, people are more likely to take advantage of you if they know you will respond to their boundary violation with mere silence. This is because silence is not a formidable deterrent to stop a boundary violation in its tracks. Speaking up for yourself or rallying allies to your cause is a much stronger response that makes the perpetrator think twice about their actions.

In addition, shame thrives in silence. When you stay silent, you deny your needs and internalize the pain from being taken advantage of. This process makes you feel worse about yourself and gets you stuck in a vicious cycle where silence and shame feed into each other.

To combat shame, recognize that setting healthy boundaries does not mean you are flawed or weak. It takes tremendous self-awareness to accept that you have reached your limits and cannot add more to your plate. It also takes great strength and courage to speak up and advocate for yourself.

It is worth noting that a fine line separates guilt from shame. Guilt can descend into shame when you internalize your shortcomings and conclude that you are inherently flawed. This is a distorted thought pattern involving the fusion of your self-worth with your actions. In other words, you are saying "I have failed. Therefore, I am a failure."

The reality is that failure does not define you. It is a universal human experience. None of us are immune to its sting. The key is to see failure as a valuable opportunity to learn and grow into a better version of yourself.

People Pleasing

A tendency to people please is another factor that interferes with boundary setting. We are social creatures who need love and connection. As a result, we are reluctant to take any risk that may disrupt relationships, even if they are unhealthy in nature.

This pattern of behavior is most evident in our interactions with parental figures. I have worked with countless physicians who had no difficulty navigating interpersonal dynamics in the professional setting. However, once it came to dealing with their parents, all bets were off.

As an example, I worked with a resident physician who was struggling with anxiety. What made her feel overwhelmed was not necessarily the grueling workload of residency or interacting with attending physicians who can be harsh in their criticisms. She also felt she was doing a great job raising a toddler during residency and maintaining a reasonable work-life balance. Navigating her relationship with her mother was the most stressful part of her life.

This physician reported that her mother had a long history of struggling with alcoholism which made her mood and behaviors erratic. She had a pattern of expecting to be the center of attention and would sabotage milestones in the physician's life. For example, her mother became intoxicated and had belligerent behavior on her wedding day which tainted the event. The physician was unsure how to handle her mother who insisted on being more involved in her child's life.

During our work together, the physician reflected on how to navigate her relationship with her mother. She certainly cared about her and wanted her to achieve sobriety. However, she also had an overriding responsibility to shield her child from her mother's erratic behaviors. How could she know that her child would be safe in her mother's presence when she had a long history of being unpredictable and destructive? Blindly succumbing to her mother's demands posed a potential risk to her child's safety. Once this risk was highlighted, the physician felt more empowered to set boundaries.

The mother initially did not respond kindly to the physician's boundaries. She employed a number of manipulative tactics to violate them. She gaslit her by claiming she was being selfish for keeping her away from her grandchild. Despite the immense pressure, the physician held her ground and did not budge to her mother's tactics. Over time, something interesting occurred. The mother realized that her tactics were not effective. Acting erratically was only validating the physician's decision to double down on her boundaries. As a result, the mother altered her approach and became more agreeable in their interactions. After all, the physician held the leverage in their relationship. She had the final say in determining how much time her mother could spend with her child.

This example shows how setting boundaries is initially hard. You are likely to experience backlash from the person who does not want your boundaries in place. Over time, boundary setting becomes easier. Once you have established the precedent, keeping boundaries in place is not as hard.

This pattern is true for many things in life. Starting any exercise routine is hard. It can be difficult to perform a squat or go for a run when you are deconditioned. It gets easier over time. Consistent practice helps you develop the necessary muscle memory, strength and endurance to perform an exercise routine more feasibly.

The same holds true for setting boundaries. With practice, you are better able to hold your ground. Emotional forces such as guilt and the need to please do not have the same impact on you. Instead of reflexively caving in to manipulative tactics you prioritize your needs over their wants.

It is worth noting that as you consistently set healthy boundaries, people start to perceive you differently. Over time, you become known as a person with firm boundaries and people are less likely to test them. Instead, they will seek someone more accommodating. It is human nature to pursue the path of least resistance and approach the person who is most likely to respond favorably to one's request.

Boundaries are an essential component of any healthy relationship. Someone who truly cares about you will honor your boundaries. They may not necessarily like them, but they will respect them and certainty not try to manipulate you into saying Yes.

One helpful tactic to overcome the tendency to people please is to realize that the quality of your decisions is not defined by how someone feels about them. Someone may be upset with you even though you made the right decision. As a clinical example, imagine you are working with a patient seeking treatment for panic attacks. They ask you to prescribe a benzodiazepine, such as Xanax, for relief. On history, you find out they suffer from alcoholism and are consuming 12 beers per day. Prescribing Xanax may satisfy your patient. It may provide temporary relief to their anxiety. They may even give you a glowing review on a patient satisfaction survey. However, it is an inappropriate treatment intervention because the concurrent use of the medication and alcohol can significantly reduce their respiratory rate and lead to mortality. As a result, declining their request is the correct decision even if they are upset with you.

You need to be comfortable with the fact that you will disappoint, and even upset, people. You cannot please everyone. Different people have competing goals, values and expectations. It is impossible to be everything for everyone. Radically accepting this undeniable reality will allow you to be intentional in how you arrive at your decisions.

Self-Reliant

As previously discussed, medicine has taught you to be stoic and self-reliant. You are skilled in putting everyone's needs ahead of your own. This mindset makes it hard to set healthy boundaries by asking for help when the need arises.

A common myth among physicians is that being self-reliant is the equivalent of never asking for help. Contrary to what you learned in your training, we are interdependent beings who rely on one another for help and support. None of us would have made it this far in our personal and professional lives without the grace of people who have helped us along the way.

As a personal example, I would not be the human being I am today without the grace of my parents who worked tirelessly to instill values in me such as empathy, kindness and service. I would not be the physician I am today without the countless mentors and professors who taught me the intricacies of medicine and how to be a doctor. On a daily basis, I rely on support staff who coordinate patient care. Finally, I could have never written this book without the support of my wife who stood firmly by my side while I wrote it.

When you ask someone for help, you are sending the message that they are trustworthy and reliable. This can make them feel good about themselves. Asking for help can also strengthen interpersonal relationships because it allows you to, at least momentarily, shed your physician façade and reveal a more vulnerable, human side which is easier to connect with.

Success does not occur in a silo. It takes a village for anyone to excel. Asking for help is nothing to be ashamed of. The key is to make a reasonable ask, express sincere gratitude for receiving help and find ways to return the favor.

Need for Control

An additional factor interfering with your ability to set healthy boundaries is your need for control. Delegating tasks is difficult because it requires you to relinquish some control. You have to rely on someone else to complete a task that you would be more than capable of completing if you had the time. This introduces an element of uncertainty. How can you be certain that someone else will complete the assigned task as well as you would?

The reality is that you have no choice but to mindfully relinquish some of your responsibilities. Refusing to delegate because of your need for control is a surefire way to have your life spiral out of control as you buckle from the collective weight of competing responsibilities.

Accept the limitations in how much control you truly have. You do not even have full control of your body. Your immune system fights off invaders without your input. Your heart beats tirelessly day and night. You go on with your daily life without commanding your liver, thyroid and kidneys to complete their important daily functions. If you have such little control over your body, how much control over other people or situations do you really have?

One of the few things you have control over is setting healthy boundaries by saying No, asking for help and delegating tasks appropriately. This starts by being honest with yourself and honoring your limits. You can't be the perfect physician, parent, spouse, son or daughter, sibling, friend, homeowner and citizen simultaneously. You have a finite amount of time, energy and resources. Being judicious in how you employ them is within your sphere of control.

Fear of Repercussion

Setting boundaries can be difficult when you fear repercussions for your behavior. This emotional barrier is quite common in medicine because its hierarchical structure creates power differentials, which make it intimidating to advocate for yourself.

As an example, I worked with an attending physician who was struggling to keep up with the frantic pace of the outpatient clinic. She would fall behind because certain patients required more time and attention than the customary 20-minute time slot would allow. To compensate, she started blocking her schedule to allow more time for complex patient encounters.

During one of our sessions, she reported her practice manager confronted her about her scheduling tactic. The manager wondered why she needed more time for certain patient encounters when no other physician in the practice took such measures. The physician felt intimidated and considered abandoning the strategy for fear of repercussions. Nevertheless, she stood her ground. She explained the rationale for her actions and how rushing through more complex cases could compromise patient care. She also reported that regularly falling behind was not fair to patients who arrived on time for their scheduled appointments.

It is worth noting that her fear of repercussions never came to reality. The practice manager approached her a number of times to question her behavior. Yet, the physician continued to prioritize her patients by giving them the time they needed. She ultimately had the final say in determining what was in their best interest.

Another noteworthy point is that other physicians in this practice started following her lead by allocating more time for complex clinical encounters. Her courage to stand her ground had a positive ripple effect on her colleagues who were inspired to modify the way they cared for patients.

In different clinical settings, people will test your boundaries because their goals are not necessarily aligned with yours. As a physician, your primary goal is to provide the best quality care to your patients. A practice manager cares about this as well. However, they also care about additional variables such as how much revenue is generated by the practice, the number of patients seen per day and maximizing patient satisfaction scores. Conflict between different parties arises because goals are not in alignment.

To cope with such conflict, recognize how much leverage you truly have. You are the expert. Many people can fill the role of your practice manager or hospital administrator. Few have the expertise and experience to care for your patients. Do not relinquish your authority or autonomy the first time you receive backlash.

It can be difficult setting boundaries if other physicians in your work environment are not engaging in this behavior. You may be hesitant to stand apart from your colleagues for fear of being labelled as difficult. What is harder to deal with is the realization that you spent years of your life and hundreds of thousands of dollars in tuition to become a physician, only to relinquish your authority and autonomy to parties in the healthcare system who do not have your medical knowledge or expertise. If other physicians choose not to advocate for themselves, this does not mean you have to follow suit. You can lead by example and role model for your colleagues how to reclaim their agency in clinical medicine.

Anxiety will always tell you not to advocate for yourself. It will zoom in on the worst-case scenario and treat it as imminent and inevitable even if it has a low probability of occurrence. It will magnify the potential repercussions of standing up for yourself.

Let's assume that your greatest fear is being fired for refusing to acquiesce to the demands of your employer. What are the odds that you will be fired considering there is a physician shortage in the U.S. that is projected to reach nearly 140,000 physicians by 2033 (3)? Also, replacing a physician comes at a tremendous cost to a healthcare system. On average, it takes 4.3 months to fill a vacant family medicine physician position and up to ten months to replace a specialist. In that time, hospitals can lose $559,000 for not having filled the family medicine position and even more for specialist positions (4). When you consider the costs associated with physician recruitment, the last thing a hospital wants to do is fire you and look for your replacement.

However, let's assume you have a streak of bad luck and the worst-case scenario comes to reality. You lose your job because you stood up for yourself. What would you do in this worst-case scenario? Could you handle it? Would you not find another job? Of course, you would. The new job may not be perfect. You may have to deal with a longer commute or a pay cut. You may even have to move to a different location. Nevertheless, you would undoubtedly get back on your feet and feel proud of yourself for having the courage to leave a toxic work environment which was taking advantage of you.

Worst-case scenarios are often difficult and intimidating. Yet, you have what it takes to navigate them. Coming to this realization reduces the fear associated with potentially facing repercussions for setting boundaries.

There are two sides to every coin. Anxiety only focuses on one side and magnifies the potential cost of setting boundaries. However, it does not give you the complete picture. It does not tell you that the actual cost of not advocating for yourself is often greater. If you never say No to others, then you will end up saying No to yourself and the people who matter most to you. You will regret this tradeoff in the long run.

Practical Tips

There are a number of emotional forces that make it difficult to set boundaries in your personal and professional life. Learning to identify and navigate these barriers is a skill that can be cultivated with consistent practice. Be patient with yourself as you work on developing this skill. A good starting point is to set boundaries with yourself by having realistic expectations of yourself. Navigating interpersonal relationships is harder when you expect yourself to always make sacrifices. It is ok to prioritize and advocate for your needs. Setting boundaries with others is not a luxury, but a necessity.

As you work on setting boundaries, start slow. You might feel more comfortable making smaller asks before jumping to larger ones. As an example, I worked with an older gentleman who worked part-time and babysat his grandchild two days per week. Though he enjoyed time with his grandchild, he started to feel taken for granted by his daughter and son-in-law. The agreement was for them to pick up their child at 4 pm, unless they had to stay late for work. In a matter of a few months, they became lax and would consistently arrive past the agreed time. The grandfather tried to stay silent to avoid a potential confrontation. However, suppressing one's thoughts and feelings does not work in the long run. The weight of the cognitive and emotional load eventually takes its toll without addressing the problem at hand (5).

To address the situation, the grandfather started slow by reminding his family they had to arrive by 4 pm, as originally agreed upon, to take their child. He warned them if they did not honor their part of the agreement then he would escalate his boundaries and not honor his part which would force them to look for alternative childcare solutions. As you can imagine, the parents started coming on time to pick up their child, though they were initially standoffish in their interactions.

Another tip to help you set boundaries is to press pause before reflexively saying Yes. In an effort to avoid difficult emotions, such as anxiety or guilt, the reflex is to give an immediate Yes when a request is made. The problem with this approach is that you will still experience difficult emotions at a later time such as resentment for reluctantly saying Yes or anxiety due to being overwhelmed with responsibilities.

It is ok to buy some time before giving an immediate answer. You may respond by saying: "Thank you for asking for my help. Let me discuss it with loved ones before I make a decision." Such a response conveys the message that you appreciate their ask, but it also impacts loved ones. As a result, you need to take them into consideration before making a decision.

Furthermore, setting boundaries can be more feasible if you have allies who are willing to support your cause. I believe this is most crucial for resident physicians who need to be very tactful in how they stand up for themselves because they have much less leverage in the hierarchical structure of medicine. Not graduating residency can derail a physician's career.

A final tip is to keep your explanations brief when setting boundaries. A simple "Thank you but No" can suffice. Offering a lengthy explanation with the reasons for declining a request can reveal your hand and be used to manipulate your No into a Yes.

Your different personal and professional roles come with a host of competing responsibilities. Setting boundaries is essential to navigate them. The reality is that saying Yes to everything is a recipe for struggling with burnout because you only have so much emotional energy, focus and time. Though it can be difficult to set boundaries due to emotional forces, you have no choice but to hone this skill. The cost of not setting boundaries is too great to ignore.

References

1. Rapp DJ, Hughey JM, Kreiner, GE. Boundary work as a buffer against burnout: evidence from healthcare workers during the COVID-19 pandemic. *Journal of Applied Psychology.* 2021;106(8):1169–1187.   https://doi.org/10.1037/apl0000951
2. Cheng Y, Chou J, Martínez RM, Fan YT, Chen C. Psychopathic traits mediate guilt-related anterior midcingulate activity under authority pressure. *Sci Rep.* 2021 Jul 21;11:14856. doi:10.1038/s41598-021-94372-5
3. New surgeon general advisory sounds alarm on health worker burnout and resignation. *U.S. Department of Health and Human Services.* May 23, 2022. Accessed November 14, 2023. https://www.hhs.gov/about/news/2022/05/23/new-surgeon-general-advisory-sounds-alarm-on-health-worker-burnout-and-resignation.html
4. Dyrda L. The cost of physician turnover. *Becker's Hospital CFO Report.* September 21, 2023. Accessed November 17, 2023. https://www.beckershospitalreview.com/finance/the-cost-of-physician-turnover.html
5. Cowan CSM, Wong SF, Le L. Rethinking the role of thought suppression in psychological models and treatment. *J Neurosci.* 2017;37(47):11293–11295. doi:10.1523/JNEUROSCI.2511-17.2017

10 In Pursuit of Perspective

It is another busy clinic day. You enter the exam room and apologize to the patient for running late. You have fallen behind and patients are becoming restless in the waiting room. You have not had a chance to write any of your notes or respond to the dozen messages from patients requesting medication refills or adjustments because the current treatment intervention is not working. It will be another late day despite skipping lunch in a futile attempt to keep up with work.

Despite your best efforts, you are having a hard time listening carefully to your patient's concerns. A variety of emotions is distracting you from the present moment. You feel anxious to rush through the encounter because of the amount of work that needs to be completed. As you think about having fallen behind, you become dejected and helpless at the realization that you always seem to run behind no matter how hard you try to avoid this. Even though your patient is speaking about a health concern, you are not present with them. Your mind has left the room which only makes you fall further behind due to being distracted.

This pattern of not being present only continues after work. You rush through dinner because you have to take your kids to extracurricular activities. While sitting in the stands, you feel antsy thinking about the notes that need to be completed. Interactions with loved ones are brief because work responsibilities are calling your name.

By the end of the day, you feel exhausted. You can barely muster enough energy to plop on the couch where you fall for the usual mind-numbing vices of consuming junk food, alcohol and Netflix reruns, while scrolling aimlessly on your phone. This pattern only makes you feel worse about yourself because you know it is not good for you. However, it is your only source of reprieve from a jam-packed day that lacks any joy or pleasure.

This pace of life is not sustainable. You wake up exhausted and dread the day ahead. Days feel the same as they bleed into each other. Instead of experiencing joy or pleasure, you feel a constant churn of overwhelm

DOI: 10.4324/9781003473923-14

as you look ahead at everything that needs to be completed. Your efforts to keep up with life's frenetic pace seem futile because you always run behind. You are living a life of quiet desperation because you know that something has to change, but don't know where to start. You feel trapped in a reality with no plausible exit. Medicine has become all-consuming and spares no time or energy for anything or anyone else.

As a physician, your reflex is to work faster and harder to keep up with increasing demands. When the going gets tough, you double down on your efforts by skipping lunch, staying later at work, cutting back on family time to write notes and abandoning every form of self-care. This approach is understandable. It helped you make it through the rigors of medical school and residency. This is how you survived 12-hour study days and 30-hour work shifts. However, it is not working for you today. Despite your herculean efforts, you are always behind, which makes you feel terrible about yourself. Work has morphed into the mythological Hydra of Lerna with no end in sight. Every time you rush to complete a task, new ones emerge to take its place.

The time has come to evolve by adopting a new approach. What helped you survive past challenges is not helping you navigate current ones. The first step is to radically accept that the current pace is not sustainable and trying to keep up is doomed to fail.

Accepting this reality helps you look at life's demands from a different lens. It also forces you to come up with different solutions that go against your instinct. Instead of working harder and rushing to keep up with unrealistic demands imposed on you, you need to slow down and be more present with a task at a particular moment. This will help you be more efficient and effective in fulfilling competing responsibilities.

The skill that can help you slow down and be less distracted is mindfulness, which is defined as the nonjudgmental awareness of the present moment. Being mindful can help you notice when your mind is wandering away and bring it back to the present moment. There is strong evidence that mindfulness practices reduce burnout in a number of work settings including healthcare (1).

When I introduce concepts such as mindfulness or boundary setting to my fellow healthcare professionals, I am often met with skepticism. Physicians often tell me that asking them to adopt these practices can feel like we are letting the healthcare system off the hook. I am asking them to add one more task to their overfilled plate without addressing the elephant in the room which is how systemic factors are contributing to their suffering. It can feel as if we are absolving hospitals, insurance companies and other parties from their culpability in the current physician mental health crisis and responsibility to address physician burnout by making healthcare more humane and less corporate.

Burnout is primarily due to systemic factors that have made it nearly impossible to be a physician without sacrificing your health and loved ones. Systemic changes are essential to protect physician health and promote patient care. Without such changes, physicians will continue to suffer. At the same time, you are responsible for navigating today's challenging climate in a healthy manner. Being equipped with the proper skills can help.

One of the concepts I teach my patients is the importance of limiting the damage that a stressor has on them. This is based on the Buddhist principle of the first and second arrow. The first arrow was shot by medicine and has hurt you. The corporatization of healthcare with an emphasis on capitalistic benchmarks puts you in a moral dilemma in which you are pressured to compromise your values to meet productivity benchmarks. The fact that you even have to advocate for yourself and your patients against this business model is evidence that healthcare has lost its moral compass.

The second arrow, which is your reaction to an external stressor, can worsen the damage sustained from the first arrow. Do not make a bad situation worse by sustaining self-inflicted injuries from a second arrow. This can occur when you allow medicine to consume every part of your life. Do not allow medicine to distract you when you take your children to extracurricular activities or when you have plans with friends. Do not think about medicine when you need to recharge your batteries on your time off. Do not allow medicine to be a source of friction between you and your partner because you are constantly consumed with work responsibilities. Do not fall for the trap of binging on junk food, alcohol and Netflix at the end of the day in search of reprieve. Being more mindful can protect you from sustaining self-inflicted injuries from the second arrow.

Being present in the moment sounds simple, but is hard to do. People spend nearly 47% of their waking hours thinking about something other than what they are doing in the present moment (2). This pattern comes at a cost. The wandering mind is unhappy, anxious and dissatisfied with life.

As an example, imagine you are folding laundry, but fantasizing about a trip to your favorite destination. This thought pattern is a source of suffering because it highlights the gap between where you are and where you wish you were. You are more likely to experience joy by focusing on the task at hand. Staying present can help you appreciate the fresh smell and warmth of laundry that just came out of the dryer. Taking your time to complete the task can be a source of pleasure. Being distracted deprives you of such simple, but satisfying, experiences.

You may wonder what is the purpose of having a wandering mind, if it is a source of emotional pain. The answer is that it was a matter of survival for our ancestors. From an evolutionary perspective, the job of your brain is not to make you happy. Its job is to protect you by looking for potential dangers. Imagine how harsh the world must have been for our ancestors, only a few thousand years ago. This is not that long ago when you consider that modern humans emerged at least 300,000 years ago (3). They had to worry about being hunted by predators. Looking into the future for potential dangers was essential to survive.

The world changes rapidly but evolution happens at a snail's pace. Consider how dramatically the world has changed during your lifetime. When you were younger, you would go to the local library and leaf through an encyclopedia to look up information. Today, you can access every bit of information from your phone. The rate of change will only increase as artificial intelligence plays a more prominent role in our lives. The human brain has not had the time to adapt to this rapid pace of change.

Unlike our ancestors, we no longer have to worry about being hunted by a lion hiding behind a bush or a lurking gator as we sip water at a pond. Today, we worry about a host of different things such as what others think of us, the well-being of loved ones, keeping up with work responsibilities, the state of the economy and world events. Though valid, worry thoughts take us away from the present moment as we drift away into hypothetical scenarios, many of which never come to fruition.

Cultivating mindfulness can help you regulate your emotions more effectively (4). Additional benefits include a reduction in anxiety levels, improvement in attention and cognitive flexibility and enjoying greater relationship satisfaction (5,6,7). Being mindful will help you make the most of the present moment, even though different work and social obligations pull you in different directions.

A less-known benefit of mindfulness is that it can help you experience more gratitude in your daily life. Findings show a significant association between mindfulness and gratitude (8). Similar to mindfulness, the practice of gratitude can help reduce burnout. A prospective study of 1,575 healthcare workers showed that practicing gratitude was associated with significant improvements in emotional exhaustion, happiness and work-life balance (9).

Gratitude, like mindfulness, is often met with skepticism. It has become synonymous with toxic positivity which refers to only looking at life's stressors from a positive lens while ignoring any difficult emotions that may be associated with them. Telling someone to only look on the bright side is dismissive because it invalidates the impact of stressors and the difficult feelings that are associated with them.

In reality, gratitude does not dismiss the difficulties you are going through or invalidate your emotions. It provides a healthy counterbalance to your brain's evolutionary tendency of looking into the future for what can go wrong. Gratitude provides a powerful reminder that your life, in its present state, has both real challenges that need to be addressed and also blessings to be appreciated.

The human brain is constantly processing vast amounts of information. To deal with this, it seeks shortcuts by looking for predictable patterns that help it rapidly make sense of the surrounding environment (10). This learning process results in automatic patterns of thinking and behaving. Imagine how bogged down you would feel if you had to think hard about daily tasks that you automatically complete such as tying your shoelaces or reading facial expressions. In an effort to simplify the learning process, the brain prefers the shortcut of thinking in absolute polarities such as black or white instead of trying to decipher different shades of gray.

Unfortunately, this pattern of thinking comes at a cost to your emotional health. For example, perfectionism stems from thinking in absolute terms. From a perfectionist's perspective, they are either perfect or a complete failure with no possibilities between these polar opposites. This makes for a suffocating way to live due to the pressure of trying to meet unrealistic standards. A healthier perspective is to recognize that you have strengths and imperfections which are potential opportunities for improvement. To be human is to have flaws.

Thinking in absolute terms also pits people against each other. It is much easier to think that someone is either completely with you or against you instead of taking a more nuanced approach where you agree on certain topics and disagree on others. This pattern of thinking is having a devastating impact on society as people from different sides of the political spectrum only focus on their differences while ignoring opportunities for cooperation and collaboration.

Gratitude can protect you from thinking in absolute terms. Substituting "all or nothing" with "and" statements opens you to perspectives that are more nuanced, and also accurate, representations of what we experience in our daily lives. Every single day comes with both joyful and painful experiences. You can feel sad and happy simultaneously about a particular event such as a dear friend leaving for greener pastures.

It can be difficult to notice the rays of sun peeking through the clouds. Once again, dissatisfaction serves an important evolutionary purpose. For our ancestors who lived in a harsher and more unpredictable environment, being satisfied could jeopardize their survival. A chronic sense of dissatisfaction provided them with a powerful motive to accumulate more food resources in anticipation of future inclement conditions. Today, this motive plays out as people accumulate more wealth, fame, power and prestige with no end in sight.

Gratitude can help you counteract your brain's evolutionary tendencies. It is easy to zoom in on your worries and focus on everything that is wrong with life. This tendency is the equivalent of focusing on the branches of a tree and noticing how crooked they are. Gratitude helps you zoom out and remember you are in the midst of a majestic forest. Changing how you view your reality with a conscious focus on blessings can have emotional and interpersonal benefits (11).

Being mindful takes practice. You cannot be mindful doing mindless things. The good news is this skill can be cultivated through consistent practice.

Here are some strategies to help you be more mindful in your daily life.

1. Check in with Your Body

Anxiety can present with different physical symptoms such as muscle tension, shallow breathing, talking faster and fidgeting. We are often unaware of how much tension our bodies hold. We experience discomfort in our upper back and neck muscles without realizing that our shoulders have been shrugged towards our ears. We become short of breath without noticing that our breathing has been shallow and rapid due to anxiety.

Mindfulness can help you be more connected with your body and aware of how emotional states affect it. Take a moment to notice your level of anxiety and how it manifests in your body. If your shoulders are shrugged towards your ears, slowly drop them to a more relaxed position. If your calves are tight, spend a few minutes stretching them. Observe your breathing rate. If your breathing is shallow and rapid, take a few slow, deep breaths. These interventions only take a few minutes but can make a big difference in reducing your overall levels of anxiety.

2. Take the Scenic Route

In our haste to keep up with competing responsibilities, we miss out on daily opportunities for pleasure and connection. Though small and seemingly mundane, these opportunities are meaningful.

As an example, I worked with a physician who would rush home after a hard day at work to get a head start on her evening to-do list revolving around childcare and domestic tasks. While working together, I asked her to consider the impact of taking the longer, scenic way home. Would adding an extra five or ten minutes to her commute negatively impact her ability to keep up with her evening responsibilities? Would anyone be upset with her for arriving home a few minutes later? Could having a few extra minutes to herself help her be more present when she arrived home?

Interestingly, she enjoyed taking the scenic route home. Slowing down to savor the scenery allowed her to process work stressors and let go of difficult feelings before arriving home. This helped her be more present with loved ones and effective in completing her evening responsibilities.

These small moments are scattered throughout the day. They may include slowing down to enjoy a meal, chatting with a colleague for a few minutes between cases, or taking pleasure in a warm shower. Though brief, these moments can have a positive impact on your day.

3. Start a Meditation Practice

Mindfulness meditation is a practice in which you train yourself to be more mindful. Starting such a practice is not complicated. Find a quiet room where you can sit comfortably for five minutes without any distractions. Close your eyes and focus on taking slow, deep breaths.

This exercise sounds simple but is difficult to execute. Your brain will resist staying in the present moment as it generates a cascade of random thoughts ranging from what needs to be completed on your to-do list to trying to solve existential matters such as the meaning of life. When you notice your brain wander away, gently bring it back to your breath.

The goal of this exercise is not necessarily to maintain your focus on the quality of your breathing for the entire duration. The goal is to notice when your brain wanders away and to bring your attention back to your breath in a nonjudgmental manner. The act of returning to the present moment is the equivalent of performing a biceps curl during an arm workout. This is when you grow your mindfulness muscle.

There are different types of meditation. Personally, I practice gratitude meditation every morning. Before I head out the door to go to work, I identify one thing that I am grateful for and spend one minute feeling gratitude. My focus may include a loved one, my health, a positive life experience, the privilege of practicing medicine, daily comforts we often take for granted or the gift of life. Focusing on such blessings helps me start the day on the right foot.

At times, my gratitude meditation focuses on tribulations I have been spared. The reality is that there are people in the world who have it much worse than you and me. Their suffering does not negate your suffering. Your pain is real and valid. However, it is important to maintain perspective by appreciating your blessings in the midst of your life's challenges.

4. Detach from Technology

Our smartphones can be addicting. We spend more time on them than we care to admit. Being present is difficult when you are attached to a phone that rings every time you get an email, text or social media notification.

In addition, just the sight of your phone is a distraction. It subconsciously triggers the urge to pick it up and look for notifications, which takes you away from the present moment.

Its distracting effects became apparent to me on a previous family vacation. I had gone for a light jog on the beach. The sight and sound of the waves gently hitting the shore along with the salty ocean breeze caressing my face made for a tranquilizing experience. I was in a state of inner peace until the moment I decided to pull my phone out of my pocket to check the time. That is when I noticed I had received a couple text messages. I found myself taken away from my tranquil surroundings as I debated whether to open and read the messages. Would I be opening Pandora's box by reading the messages? There was a moment of real tension as I briefly deliberated about what to do. Ultimately, I decided to return to the present moment and check the messages at the end of my run. Though brief, this experience demonstrates the distracting effect of our phones. They can disrupt even the most serene setting.

Set boundaries with your smartphone. If you do not want to be distracted by it, leave it in a different room to reduce the temptation to check it. I personally leave my phone in our mudroom when I arrive home. Leaving the phone in a different room creates a protective barrier that helps me be present with loved ones.

If you need to keep your phone in your vicinity, press pause before reflexively reaching for it. Notice how you feel when you have the urge to reach for it. Perhaps you are trying to change an unpleasant emotional state such as boredom or anxiety. Take a moment to identify alternative ways of coping.

5. Journal

The brain is a master storyteller. It tells us stories that we automatically accept, even if they are not necessarily accurate.

Our pattern of thinking can make us vulnerable to difficulties with depression and anxiety. It can be difficult to identify such patterns as they elude our consciousness in our wandering minds. Writing down your thoughts in a journaling exercise allows you to mobilize your sensory system when looking for cognitive errors. You can see the thought which has been troubling you. It can no longer escape your awareness because it is contained in written form.

Black-or-white thinking is an example of a cognitive distortion associated with depression and anxiety. Additional examples include jumping to premature conclusions without having all the facts, treating the worst-case scenario as imminent even if it has a low probability of occurrence, blaming yourself for things that are not your fault, overgeneralizing an isolated incident and magnifying the negative while ignoring the positive.

Grab a pen and paper to write your thoughts and feelings about different stressors. Focus on what you can do to address them. Try to identify cognitive distortions in the way you perceive them and alternative ways of looking at them.

6. Spend Time in Nature

There is something both soothing and energizing about spending time in nature. It is awe-inspiring to be exposed to nature's innate grandeur, majesty and beauty, a sharp contrast to the pollution, waste and noise caused by human encroachment.

Allowing your senses to be bathed by the sounds, smells and sights of nature can enhance mindful awareness (12). Time slows down when you remove yourself from the daily hustle and immerse yourself in nature. Being exposed to nature's vastness is an important reminder of our place in the world. At the end of the day, each one of us is a finite speck. Life has existed before our arrival on this planet and will continue after our demise.

Coming to this realization is liberating. It gives you permission to accept your rightful place on this planet and not overextend yourself beyond it. You do not have to carry the burdens of the world on your shoulders, nor are you responsible for curing an entire healthcare system plagued by a host of systemic factors beyond your control. Simply take the time to appreciate the gift of life and make the most of it by having a positive ripple effect on the people you can touch with your words and actions.

In summary, practicing mindfulness and gratitude can help you gain a new perspective which can reduce burnout, improve your mood and positively impact your interpersonal relationships. These practices can help you navigate more effectively the host of systemic factors that interfere with your ability to practice medicine.

References

1. Luken M, Sammons A. Systematic review of mindfulness practice for reducing job burnout. *Am J Occup Ther.* 2016;70(2):7002250020p1-7002250020p10. doi:10.5014/ajot.2016.016956
2. Killingsworth MA, Gilbert DT. A wandering mind is an unhappy mind. *Science.* 2010;330(6006):932. doi:10.1126/science.1192439
3. Handwerk B. An evolutionary timeline of homo sapiens. *Smithsonian Magazine.* February 2, 2021. Accessed November 23, 2023. https://www.smithsonianmag.com/science-nature/essential-timeline-understanding-evolution-homo-sapiens-180976807/
4. Farb NA, Anderson AK, Mayberg H, Bean J, McKeon D, Segal ZV. Minding one's emotions: mindfulness training alters the neural expression of sadness [published correction appears in *Emotion*, 2010 Apr;10(2):215]. *Emotion.* 2010;10(1):25–33. doi:10.1037/a0017151

5. Hofmann SG, Sawyer AT, Witt AA, Oh D. The effect of mindfulness-based therapy on anxiety and depression: a meta-analytic review. *J Consult Clin Psychol*. 2010;78(2):169–183. doi:10.1037/a0018555

6. Moore A, Malinowski P. Meditation, mindfulness and cognitive flexibility. *Conscious Cogn*. 2009;18(1):176–186. doi:10.1016/j.concog.2008.12.008

7. Barnes S, Brown KW, Krusemark E, Campbell WK, Rogge RD. The role of mindfulness in romantic relationship satisfaction and responses to relationship stress. *J Marital Fam Ther*. 2007;33(4):482–500. doi:10.1111/j.1752-0606.2007.00033.x

8. Swickert R, Bailey E, Hittner J, et al. The meditational roles of gratitude and perceived support in explaining the relationship between mindfulness and mood. *J Happiness Stud*. 2019;20:815–828. https://doi.org/10.1007/s10902-017-9952-0

9. Adair KC, Rodriguez-Homs LG, Masoud S, Mosca PJ, Sexton JB. Gratitude at work: prospective cohort study of a web-based, single-exposure well-being intervention for health care workers. *J Med Internet Res*. 2020;22(5):e15562. doi:10.2196/15562

10. Konovalov A, Krajbich I. Neurocomputational dynamics of sequence learning. *Neuron*. 2018;98(6):1282–1293. https://doi.org/10.1016/j.neuron.2018.05.013

11. Emmons RA, McCullough ME. Counting blessings versus burdens: an experimental investigation of gratitude and subjective well-being in daily life. *Journal of Personality and Social Psychology*. 2003;84(2):377–389. https://doi.org/10.1037/0022-3514.84.2.377

12. Van Gordon W, Shonin E, Richardson M. Mindfulness and nature. *Mindfulness*. 2018;9:1655–1658. https://doi.org/10.1007/s12671-018-0883-6

11 Tame Your Inner Critic

We are all familiar with the following scenario. We make an innocent mistake and start berating ourselves by saying things such as:

"I am such an idiot. I can't believe I screwed up."

"What's wrong with me? How could I get that wrong?"

"I am such a failure. How did I even become a physician?"

These phrases are a PG version of what I commonly hear from physicians for even the most miniscule mistake. You would never speak like that to your pets, let alone another human being. But when it comes to yourself, the gloves are off. Your Inner Critic lashes out with no mercy.

Why do we talk to ourselves with such harshness? According to Freud, this results from having a superego, the part of our three-fold personality structure which serves as our conscience. It represents our highest values and orients our actions towards them. Actions that fall below this standard are met with criticism and prohibition (1).

Developed early in childhood, the superego stems from the internalized voice of parental figures who guide a child's actions by teaching them right from wrong. Tactics to change behaviors include positively reinforcing good behavior and punishing undesirable behavior. The superego is further reinforced by social institutions that guide behavior towards ideals such as the education system and organized religion.

Superego

The superego serves important functions. It is the voice you hear when facing temptations. This voice tells you not to eat that extra cookie because it is not good for you and to go to bed at an appropriate time because you have to work the following day. Throughout your academic studies, this voice urged you to skip a night out with friends because you had to

DOI: 10.4324/9781003473923-15

study for an upcoming exam. It helped you endure the hardships of medical school and residency training by delaying gratification in pursuit of a higher ideal.

In addition to prohibiting temptations, your superego gives rise to your Inner Critic who punishes you for not heeding its warnings. You have felt a combination of painful emotions such as anxiety, sadness and guilt every time your Inner Critic lashed out because your actions failed to meet expectations. This is a painful experience that is seared in your emotional memory. It prompts you to press pause and consider the consequences of your actions. Resisting primitive impulses would be exponentially harder without the threat of being disciplined.

To some degree, your Inner Critic helps you be a better version of yourself. Relying primarily on the tactic of punishment, it orients your actions towards ideals such as selflessness, integrity, honesty and loyalty by stopping questionable behaviors in their tracks. Even in the absence of external consequences, the thought of engaging in a questionable behavior can trigger feelings of guilt which make you think twice before acting (2). Like an invisible electric fence that warns your pet not to leave the premises of your property, your Inner Critic warns you not to proceed by jolting you.

Your superego also promotes social cohesion. Without it, you would blindly follow selfish impulses without any regard for their impact on others. Our internal and external worlds would disintegrate into utter chaos if safety, love and connection took a back seat to everyone's guilty pleasures.

The problem is not the presence of an Inner Critic or superego. Orienting your behavior towards an ideal target comes with individual and social benefits. The problem is your Inner Critic is excessively harsh and punitive when you fail to meet the target. It has morphed into a ruthless tyrant who beats you mercilessly for every miniscule deviation from self-imposed and societal standards. The punishment is often excessive and disproportionate to the crime.

Perfectionism and the Superego

Perfectionism is often an attempt to avoid painful feelings that stem from not meeting the demands of a harsh superego (3). This approach comes at a great cost. One of the downfalls of perfectionism is having a narrow definition of success and a broad definition of failure. You have raised the target for success to such heights that being a physician is no longer considered an achievement, despite the tremendous sacrifices you made to achieve this goal.

At the same time, any deviation from perfection is considered a failure and triggers your Inner Critic to unleash severe punishment. When you raise your bar of expectations to extreme heights, you also broaden your definition of failure to the point that even outstanding work is met with disappointment. I have worked with medical students who experienced tremendous angst and despair because they earned a B on an exam. I have also worked with medical students who thought their world was going to crash because their score on the USMLE Step exam, though satisfactory, was not as high as they had hoped for. In both scenarios, the students were well on their way to materializing their dreams of becoming physicians. However, their perfectionism had clouded their perspective on their academic performance.

Resident physicians are not exempt from the distorting effects of perfectionism. I have treated residents who were distraught to not receive a perfect score on their performance reviews. They interpreted feedback from supervising attendings as a personal failing rather than an opportunity for self-improvement. I often remind them there is a reason their training lasts for 3–7 years depending on their specialty. There would be no purpose to such vigorous training if it was not necessary to become attending physicians.

Perfectionism is a rigged game because the outcome is predetermined. You will inevitably suffer. Either you break your back trying to be perfect or suffer the wrath of your Inner Critic for failing to be perfect. The paradox of perfectionism is that it increases the odds you will be punished by your Inner Critic which is what you are trying to avoid in the first place by pursuing perfection. Blurring the definitions of success and failure makes for a brutal way to live life. It is no surprise that perfectionism is associated with burnout and a host of emotional difficulties (4).

Perfectionism and Fear of Failure

Perfectionists fear failure because the subsequent punishment from their Inner Critic is painful. As a result, they avoid situations with a high likelihood of failure. Though understandable, such an approach ultimately trains your brain to be more fearful of failure, which can negatively impact your ability to face life's challenges.

As an example, I worked with a resident who was suffering from debilitating anxiety in anticipation of her upcoming Intensive Care rotation. This was a high-performing individual who had made a positive impression on her supervising physicians and peers with her knowledge and work ethic. Nevertheless, she was experiencing anxiety difficulties in the form of sleep disturbances, irritability, tension headaches and stomach discomfort leading up to the rotation.

During our work together, we explored the source of her anxiety. She was not worried about working long hours during the rotation or the medical complexity of the cases. After all, she had the necessary work ethic and clinical knowledge to care for patients in the Intensive Care Unit. Rather, her anxiety stemmed from the fear of a patient dying under her care. This was her definition of failure and the possibility of such an outcome caused her tremendous distress. She interpreted it as a personal indictment and evidence that she was not a competent resident.

As part of exposure therapy, I asked her to imagine her reaction if a patient passed away even though she had implemented appropriate treatment interventions. She reported that she would consider ending her residency training prematurely because such a failure would mean she was unworthy to be a physician.

Her spike in anxiety is not surprising when you consider the cruelty of her Inner Critic. Not only was she burdened by the weight of unrealistic expectations, the punishment for not meeting them was cataclysmic. She was willing to throw away years of training over an outcome that was not an accurate reflection of her abilities as a physician.

One of the goals of our work was to tame her perfectionism by recalibrating self-imposed expectations. I wanted her to redefine failure by focusing more on the process that led to clinical outcomes. Even though the pursuit of the perfect outcome helped her make it this far in her training, it was currently coming at a cost to her mental health. This is because practicing medicine is not the same as taking an exam. If you study hard and know the material for an exam, you are likely to have the positive outcome of earning a high score. This is not necessarily the case in medicine. You can make the correct medical interventions based on sound clinical judgment and still experience the negative outcome of a patient experiencing a side effect, staying ill or even dying. The human body is much more complex than any exam you have ever taken.

As we worked together, I helped her realize that she did not have complete control over the clinical outcome of her ICU patients. Fragile, medically-compromised patients die despite providing appropriate medical interventions. Instead of focusing solely on outcomes, I asked her to focus on the process of practicing medicine. She could use her anxiety as fuel to study for the upcoming rotation. By preparing to the best of her ability both prior to and during the rotation, she could rest assured that she was doing the very best for her patients regardless of how they responded to her treatment interventions.

Self-Sabotage

Sometimes the punishment from the Inner Critic is subtle. As another example, I worked with a resident struggling with depression and anxiety.

She felt lonely and wanted to connect with peers. However, she kept to herself and skipped get-togethers because she thought her colleagues did not like her.

This resident also suffered from imposter syndrome. Even though she had received positive performance reviews from supervising attending physicians, she viewed herself as less skilled compared to her colleagues.

Her difficulties would come to the surface every time she had to attend weekly noon conference. She dreaded attending the conference for fear of being asked questions by supervising physicians that would reveal her lack of knowledge. She experienced debilitating panic attacks on the days of the conference and wished she could skip it.

During our work together, I asked her to consider whether her views of herself as a physician were based on reality or unfair self-imposed expectations. By checking the facts, such as performance reviews, it became apparent that her perceptions were not based on objective data, but stemmed from trying to be perfect to appease an overly harsh Inner Critic.

In addition, we explored her perception of what her colleagues thought of her. She denied having any negative interactions or conflicts with them. On a number of occasions, they had invited her to social events but she had declined. It is true and understandable that her colleagues had stopped inviting her after she had declined a number of invitations. One can endure only so many rejections before they eventually stop reaching out. However, their change in behavior was not evidence they thought poorly of her. A more likely scenario was that they were honoring her boundaries and giving her space.

This resident yearned for meaningful interpersonal relationships, which would have done wonders for her difficulties with depression and anxiety. However, she acted in a paradoxical way that kept people at arm's length. She was projecting her perception of herself onto other people. She did not think highly of herself and assumed that others had a similar opinion of her. This was her form of self-sabotage. By pushing people away, she deprived herself of the connections she craved the most.

Her silence during noon conference represented another form of self-sabotage. Staying silent prevented supervising physicians from observing her depth and breadth of medical knowledge. This approach could have backfired if supervisors started to question what was hiding behind her silence. Based on my clinical experience, silence among residents is often misinterpreted by supervising physicians as a lack of knowledge. They fail to consider the emotional forces that can lead to this presentation.

These examples illustrate how a harsh Inner Critic can lead to unfair and disproportionate self-imposed punishment. Perhaps there were times you were punished unfairly or criticized harshly by parental figures for the slightest shortcomings. In an attempt to mitigate further repercussions from your parents, you developed a tyrannical Inner Critic who carried out the punishment for them. In a way, your Inner Critic protected you from your own parents.

Taming your Inner Critic is hard because they have accompanied you the majority of your life. There is comfort in the familiar even if it comes at a cost. You might believe that having a harsh Inner Critic makes you a better physician. Having them hover over your shoulders with a whip in hand can be a powerful deterrent to cutting corners and not fully applying yourself. As a result, it may feel uncomfortable, even scary, to let go or change this familiar figure.

I would argue that you have made it this far despite your Inner Critic. Having a ruthless tyrant who cruelly tears you apart for the slightest short-coming is preventing you from reaching your fullest potential. It makes your life oppressing because you walk on eggshells fearing the next lashing. You would never employ such a suffocating strategy to inspire positive change in your children, spouse, friends or patients. You would never berate your child for getting a B on an exam or punish your patients for experiencing difficulties with managing a health condition. Why is it ok that you treat yourself any differently?

Having a harsh Inner Critic makes you prone to mental health difficul-ties. A systematic review of prospective studies found that self-criticism in a harsh and punitive manner is associated with subsequent symptoms of depression (5). It represents a form of aggression directed inwardly which is known to contribute to depressive features (6). Constantly punishing your-self for the slightest deviation from perfection can have devastating effects on your self-worth.

You are in a relationship with yourself 24/7. You talk to yourself. You think about yourself. You criticize yourself for your shortcomings and, hopefully, give yourself a pat on the back for a job well done. Cultivating a healthy relationship with yourself is an essential antidote to burnout and mental health difficulties. One of the best ways to achieve this is by taming your Inner Critic.

In addition, your relationship with yourself has a profound impact on your interactions with others. How you interact with others is a projection of how you view yourself. For example, having a negative view of yourself makes you prone to high levels of social anxiety (7). This is because you per-ceive yourself as lacking which manifests as anxiety in social interactions. When you do not hold a high opinion of yourself, you assume that others view you in a similar manner.

The goal is not necessarily to eliminate your Inner Critic, but to tame them into being kinder and more compassionate. You want your Inner Critic to be fair when evaluating you and to deliver constructive criticism that is proportionate to the shortcoming. This shift is essential to improve your relationship with yourself and others. Here are three steps to help you with this transition.

Mindfulness

We all have a voice in our heads. No, you do not have schizophrenia and are not hallucinating. This voice represents the superego and is a stream of consciousness that rarely stops talking. If you pay close attention, you can hear what it has to say.

As you observe the voice, notice it has different characteristics. Depending on your emotional state, its volume, pitch and tone may change. The voice may grow louder when you are angry, depressed or under stress. It may sound more soothing when you feel relaxed. The voice also comes with a message that follows predictable patterns. For example, it might scream at you and call you worthless, stupid or dumb after making a mistake. It may call you lazy in a condescending tone every time you want to take a break.

Observing the voice in a non-judgmental manner is the first step to taming your Inner Critic. This mindfulness exercise creates separation between you and the voice. You (the Subject) are paying attention to what the voice (the Object) is saying.

Your Inner Critic is a master storyteller who influences your thoughts, emotions and behaviors. You are often so intertwined with your Inner Critic that you blindly accept their words as factual. The ability to create distance and observe what they are saying can help you intervene to stop your Inner Critic in its tracks. As you become more mindful, you will be more proficient in detecting the attacks earlier and stopping them sooner. You could potentially even notice when your Inner Critic is about to strike and take proactive measures to stop their attack before it ever occurs.

Self-Compassion

The second step to taming your Inner Critic is to practice self-compassion. Evidence shows it can enhance well-being and reduce burnout for healthcare professionals (8).

According to Kristin Neff, PhD, a pioneer on the subject, self-compassion is the process of being compassionate with yourself. It entails giving yourself grace when you make a mistake. When you experience the sting of failure, do not ignore the pain. This approach only intensifies it. Instead, acknowledge the pain and mobilize healthy coping strategies to comfort yourself. Being kind to yourself is an essential feature of self-compassion.

Practicing self-compassion can help turn your Inner Critic into a kinder and more gentle voice. As you search for this voice, imagine a loved one is walking in your shoes. Perhaps they scored poorly on a standardized exam or made a miniscule clinical mistake. How would you talk to them in such a scenario? Would you berate them at their lowest point or give them grace?

The way you would speak to a loved one is the blueprint for practicing self-compassion. You need to speak to yourself with the same words, tone, pitch and volume. If you are being harder on yourself than others, then you are not being fair because of the double standard in how you treat yourself.

An additional component of self-compassion is the recognition that having an Inner Critic is part of the human condition (9). Failure can be an isolating experience when you feel like the only one who messes up. Feeling alone only exacerbates your pain while providing fertile soil for shame to cast its agonizing spell on you. In reality, to err is to be human. There is no human being who has not experienced the sting of failure or the urge to punish themselves for their shortcomings. There is comfort in recognizing that self-criticism is a universal human experience.

The key is to view failure as an essential ingredient for personal growth rather than a personal indictment. It is a valuable learning experience that brings you one step closer to your individual goals. I would argue that if you have not experienced any recent failures, then you are not challenging yourself sufficiently, which is a failure in itself. Playing it safe is often a disguise to avoid the sting of failure. Despite its protective function, this approach is keeping you stagnant in your current reality.

Reflecting on your journey to become a physician makes this lesson clear. Applying to medical school was a calculated risk. You took on student loans and delayed your earning potential to become a physician. You achieved this goal by betting on yourself. If you are suffering from burnout because medicine has not turned into the career you had envisioned, you will need to tap into the same mindset to change your current predicament. Perhaps, you are stuck in a job that is deeply dissatisfying because demanding hospital administrators have pushed you to your limits. To address this problem, you need to take the same leap of faith as when you decided to enter medical school. You need to bet on yourself and believe that you deserve to be treated better by advocating for yourself. If your efforts to set boundaries with your current employer reach a dead end, then you need to take the calculated risk of exploring different employment options that are more aligned with your values and lifestyle. Not taking any action to change your current reality is a failure that is destined to keep you stuck in the same painful reality.

Self-compassion can help you have a healthier relationship with failure. Be patient and compassionate with yourself as you work on this because you are trying to mold thought and behavioral patterns that are deeply rooted in your childhood and reinforced throughout the years. Your Inner

Critic has sat on their throne for decades. They will not relinquish it without putting up a fight.

Be patient with yourself. It will take time to tame your Inner Critic. I have worked with physicians who would criticize themselves for not developing self-compassion fast enough. In other words, they were hard on themselves for being hard on themselves. This vicious cycle only made it exponentially harder to dethrone their Inner Critic.

On a practical level, you can be more compassionate with yourself by writing down encouraging and supportive mantras that you can frequently refer to. Keep these mantras easily accessible by placing them in visible areas such as your bathroom mirror or nightstand. Read them daily. It is the repetition of new information that makes it second nature. This was the case when you had to memorize the brachial plexus or the circle of Willis in medical school. Learning mental health concepts and integrating them in your life is no different.

You can also increase your level of self-compassion by providing yourself physical comfort. Examples include literally giving yourself a pat on the back or going for a walk when you feel hurt by your Inner Critic.

Give Yourself Credit

Criticism is only one method to modify behavior. Another one is to reinforce behavior by giving yourself honest credit for a job well done.

Giving yourself a pat on the back may feel uncomfortable when you have only relied on criticism to raise your standards. The imbalance between criticism and credit is further proof that your Inner Critic is overly harsh and having a negative effect on your perception of yourself. If you are going to criticize yourself for your shortcomings, it is only fair that you give yourself credit for your victories.

As an exercise, take a moment to think about the patients you saw on a recent clinic day and how you felt by the end of it. Some of the patients were happy to see you and grateful for the care you provided. Taking care of them was a pleasant experience. However, these positive encounters are often overshadowed by more challenging ones in which patients were dissatisfied with you. They might have been unhappy because you were running late for their appointment or your treatment interventions were ineffective. These challenging encounters have a greater impact on your perception of the day, even if they are outnumbered by more positive ones. Superimpose systemic factors disrupting your workflow and it is evident how you would have a negative perception of your workday. Repeatedly stacking such days one on top of the other will inevitably lead any physician down the path to burnout.

Reflecting on difficult clinical encounters with curiosity and compassion is important to identify and address potential areas for improvement. However, it is equally important that these cases do not define the entirety of your day because there are many patients who appreciate you for the care you provide them. If you find yourself fixating only on challenging cases and neglecting more positives ones, then your perception of the day is being influenced by your Inner Critic.

Make it a habit to give yourself a pat on the back for the patients you helped. Notice patients who appreciate everything you have done for them. Recognizing the victories is important to overcome the cognitive distortion of mental filtering and have a more integrated and accurate view of your day. On a daily basis, we encounter a variety of patients with different temperaments, perspectives and expectations. It is important that we show up and do our best to help everyone who comes through our doors. The ability to do this, while navigating systemic factors that interfere with patient care, takes tremendous strength and resilience. This is an achievement that deserves to be acknowledged.

In summary, your Inner Critic is often overly harsh when trying to orient your behavior towards higher standards. This can make you prone to burnout and other emotional difficulties. You can tame your Inner Critic by being more mindful, practicing self-compassion and recognizing a job well done.

References

1. Weiss H. A brief history of the super-ego with an introduction to three papers. *The International Journal of Psychoanalysis*. 2020;101(4):724–734. https://doi.org/10.1080/00207578.2020.1796073
2. Meyer WS. Therapy of the conscience: technical recommendations for working on the harsh superego of the patient. *Clinical Social Work Journal*. 1998;26:353–368. https://doi.org/10.1023/A:1022821903579
3. Sorotzkin, B. The quest for perfection: avoiding guilt or avoiding shame? *Psychotherapy: Theory, Research, Practice, Training*. 1985;22(3):564–571. https://doi.org/10.1037/h0085541
4. Hill AP, Curran T. Multidimensional perfectionism and burnout: a meta-analysis. *Personality and Social Psychology Review*. 2016;20(3):269–288. https://doi.org/10.1177/1088868315596286
5. McIntyre R, Smith P, Rimes KA. The role of self-criticism in common mental health difficulties in students: a systematic review of prospective studies. *Mental Health & Prevention*. 2018;10:13–27. https://doi.org/10.1016/j.mhp.2018.02.003
6. Haddad SK, Reiss D, Spotts EL, Ganiban J, Lichtenstein P, Neiderhiser JM. Depression and internally directed aggression: genetic and environmental contributions. *J Am Psychoanal Assoc*. 2008;56(2):515–550. doi:10.1177/0003065108319727

7. Hulme N, Hirsch C, Stopa L. Images of the self and self-esteem: do positive self-images improve self-esteem in social anxiety? *Cogn Behav Ther*. 2012;41(2):163–173. doi:10.1080/16506073.2012.664557

8. Neff KD, Knox MC, Long P, Gregory K. Caring for others without losing yourself: an adaptation of the mindful self-compassion program for healthcare communities. *J Clin Psychol*. 2020;76(9):1543–1562. doi:10.1002/jclp.23007.

9. Neff KD. *Self-compassion: the proven power of being kind to yourself*. HarperCollins Publishers. 2011.

12 Create Your Purpose

Imagine eating dinner when you notice dull abdominal discomfort. At first, you might attribute the ache to what you just ate or coming down with a GI bug. You assume that you will feel better in a matter of days.

Unfortunately, the pain lingers longer than anticipated. Lying down seems to worsen it. You feel unusually tired and are losing weight due to a reduction in appetite. The combination of symptoms makes your antenna go up that something is off. You reluctantly visit your family doctor for a work up.

After a few days, your physician calls you to go over the results. You are stunned to hear that imaging shows a mass on your pancreas that is suspicious for cancer. What started as routine abdominal discomfort during dinner has turned into a serious threat to your very existence.

This scenario may sound farfetched. You might be banking on a long life ahead because you are blessed with good health. However, you know better. As a physician, you have been exposed to your fair share of unexpected human tragedies that highlight the fragility of life. It can be terrifying to imagine ending up in the same dire situation as your patients. It is far easier to be in denial and assume you have many healthy years ahead. I hope this is truly the case for you. However, the reality is your life can change in the blink of an eye.

You have feelings about your mortality. Your defense mechanisms do not make them go away. It is important to acknowledge these feelings because they can affect different aspects of your life including the way you practice medicine. A study found that death anxiety impacts the way physicians deliver news of an unexpected patient death (1).

Talking about death can feel contrary to the ethos of medicine which teaches us how to extend life by intervening when something goes wrong with the human body and mind. The ability to stabilize patients in critical condition or halt the progression of different ailments may give you a false sense of invincibility. However, your medical training does not make you

DOI: 10.4324/9781003473923-16

exempt from universal threats to one's existence such as illness, disability and death. A discussion of such matters is essential to uncover another evidence-based antidote to burnout.

Death serves important functions. On a global scale, our planet would be ravaged if humans were immortal. It would not be able to support a population in the hundreds of billions. The sheer volume of humans would deplete the planet's resources and overrun it with waste and pollution. Violence would erupt as people would fight amongst themselves for scarce resources. When considering the impact of immortality on the global eco-system, I am happy to take my turn and face the same fate as everyone else.

However, on an individual level, your mortality adds a sense of urgency to your life. Living forever would eliminate the need to take imme-diate action. You could indefinitely delay the pursuit of personal goals if tomorrow was always guaranteed. Scarcity is the catalyst that motivates you to take action and make the most of your finite time on this earth.

Your inevitable demise also inspires self-reflection. Thinking about the finality of your life raises two important questions. The first is to make sense of your existence by assigning meaning to it. The second is to figure out what to do during your lifetime by determining the purpose of your life.

If you find these questions overwhelming, recognize you are not alone. A survey of U.S. adults revealed that 36% of them had not found their pur-pose in life and 91% of them had experienced purpose anxiety at some point in their lives (2). Experiencing anxiety is completely understandable when you consider the magnitude of these questions. Trying to determine your life's purpose means you are seeking a "central, self-organizing life aim that organizes and stimulates goals, manages behaviors and provides a sense of meaning" (3). Your purpose serves as the compass that determines how to allocate your finite personal resources.

Though important, answering these questions is not sufficient. Once you determine your purpose in life, you need to bring it to fruition. This is quite challenging because competing work, family and social responsi-bilities can steer you off course. It can be quite painful to identify but not materialize your purpose in life. In the words of Henry David Thoreau, the majority of people "lead lives of quiet desperation. What is called resigna-tion is confirmed desperation" (4).

You may have quietly resigned to this reality and given up on fulfilling your life's purpose. Settling for the status quo may seem easier than taking the necessary action to change your life's trajectory. However, such resig-nation comes at a cost to your mental health. A meta-analysis of 66,468 participants found that greater purpose in life was significantly associated with lower levels of depression and anxiety (5).

Not fulfilling your purpose in life also comes at a cost to your phys-ical health. A prospective study found that not having a sense of ikigai, a

Japanese term for purpose in life, was associated with an increased risk of mortality irrespective of socioeconomic factors, psychological factors, lifestyle habits and history of illness (6).

Finding meaning is a powerful antidote to burnout. In a study of 465 academic physicians, the prevalence of burnout was affected by the amount of time participants spent working on the activity they found most meaningful. In particular, those who spent less than 20% of their time on this activity had significantly higher rates of burnout. The amount of time spent on the most meaningful activity was a stronger predictor of burnout than the number of hours worked per week, the physician's age and their specialty (7).

The cost for not fulfilling your purpose in life is cataclysmic. It extends beyond health problems and professional burnout. It will haunt you all the way to your death bed. In her book titled *The Top Five Regrets of the Dying, A Life Transformed by the Dearly Departing,* Bronnie Ware, an Australian nurse who spent years working in palliative care, recorded the top regrets of the dying. The first one is: "I wish I'd had the courage to live a life true to myself, not the life others expected of me" (8).

You entered medicine with the purest intentions. Medicine was a calling to serve people by alleviating their pain and suffering. Fulfilling this mission was supposed to be a major source of meaning and purpose in your life. You endured tremendous sacrifices to become a physician believing it would ultimately be worth it.

Unfortunately, you suffer deep moral injury because medicine lacks the meaning and purpose you had envisioned. Going into work has become a daily grind because the sacred patient-physician relationship has been tarnished by documentation requirements, prior authorization forms and performance benchmarks that prioritize profits over patient care. Being a physician no longer feels like a meaningful endeavor, but more like being a worker on a conveyer belt who rushes through patient encounters to satisfy the demands of administrators. Practicing medicine on such terms deprives it of purpose and meaning.

There is a strong urge to give up on your calling. It feels demoralizing when you realize that you worked so hard for so long to develop the necessary clinical skills to practice medicine only to have systemic factors, that are beyond your control, undermine them and prevent you from delivering the highest quality care. Interestingly, shutting down is the default response when you are repeatedly exposed to a stressor. This response is termed learned helplessness, though there is nothing learned about it. It is an automatic response that is mediated by the serotonergic activity of the dorsal raphe nucleus (9). It is in your DNA to feel helpless and shut down in response to a chronic stressor.

Giving up might feel easier than fighting back to derive purpose and meaning from your profession. After all, the systemic factors plaguing medicine are much bigger than you. They will continue to interfere with patient care no matter how hard you fight back.

This is a dangerous way of thinking. You need to avoid the trap of learned helplessness because it does not serve you. A life without purpose only sets you up for a woeful future plagued by health problems, burnout and regrets on your death bed. You have to fight back against such a fate. You deserve better. You did not sacrifice the best years of your life to become a physician only to fall for such a somber outcome.

You will die. You cannot escape your inevitable demise. However, you can escape being tormented with regrets on your death bed by having lived a purposeful and meaningful life.

You have more authority, autonomy and ability than you realize. You may have a hard time seeing this because you have a distorted view of reality. Systemic factors have gaslit you into believing that you are responsible for your suffering. In response to the burnout epidemic, hospital leadership may require you to attend a wellness lecture on your time off to show you different ways to be more resilient. Such generic responses to your plight are a form of gaslighting because they place the entire onus of your suffering solely on you without acknowledging the persistent and critical role that systemic factors play. Within this context, interventions that could help you overcome burnout are converted by the system into tactics that imply you are inadequate and should be doing more to handle the demands of practicing clinical medicine. Their underlying message is "If you only practiced more mindfulness, exercised more often and ate more avocados, you would be more resilient to handle the workload." Such tactics do not promote physician wellness. On the contrary, they use physician wellness as a disguise to manipulate you into working to the point of exhaustion to meet their objectives.

You need to resist the default response of shutting down. Take action to rise above the systemic factors that have tarnished healthcare. This starts by rediscovering your purpose in life. Engaging in a life-crafting intervention can help you identify what is important to you and formulate plans to achieve your goals. Life-crafting is defined as

> a process in which people actively reflect on their present and future life, set goals for important areas of life – social, career, and leisure time – and, if required, make concrete plans and undertake actions to change these areas in a way that is more congruent with their values and wishes. (10)

The overall process of writing about one's personal goals and being specific in what strategies will be employed for attaining them can lead to an improvement in performance (11).

Here are potential components of such an intervention with a sample of thought-provoking questions to identify sources of purpose in your life. The following list is not exhaustive, but can serve as a framework to reflect on your life. Modify it as you see fit.

A. Values
    a. What do I stand for?
    b. What am I passionate about?
    c. What qualities do I admire in others?
    d. How do I want to be remembered when I die?
    e. If I only had one year left to live, how would I live my life differently?
    f. If I were to die today, would I die with any regrets? What changes can I make to avoid them?

B. Career
    a. Why did I enter medicine?
    b. How much meaning do I derive from my current job?
    c. What steps can I take to derive more meaning from my current job?
    d. Are there other opportunities in clinical medicine that I would find more fulfilling?
    e. Have I recently explored my career options? If so, what opportunities have spiked my interest? Do I want to apply for them? What is holding me back from exploring them?

C. Relationships
    a. How satisfied am I with the quality of my closest relationships? Do I need to take steps to strengthen these bonds?
    b. How satisfied am I with the quantity of my relationships? Do I want more people in my life? If so, how could I cultivate more relationships?
    c. Which relationships energize me? How can I spend more time with these individuals?
    d. Which relationships deplete me? How can I spend less time with these individuals?

D. Interests
    a. What interests did I enjoy when I was younger?
    b. What are some of my interests outside of medicine?
    c. Which activities make time fly because I thoroughly enjoy them?
    d. How much time do I allocate to these activities on a weekly basis?
    e. Do I need to allocate more time to these activities? If so, how can I achieve this?

E. Self-Care
  a. What activities do I engage in to promote my physical and mental health? How do I feel after engaging in these activities?
  b. How much time do I spend on these activities per day? Per week?
  c. How can I spend more time on these activities?
  d. What unhealthy habits do I engage in? How do I feel afterwards?
  e. What are my triggers for these unhealthy habits?
  f. What emotions am I trying to mask when I engage in unhealthy habits? Examples can include trying to cope with feelings of anxiety, low mood or even boredom.
  g. Can I substitute these unhealthy habits with healthier ones to achieve the same results?

Write down your answers to these questions. Return to them periodically, every 1–3 months, to monitor your progress.

Engaging in this thought-provoking activity can be painful. You might be reluctant to answer these questions because it feels like rubbing salt on a wound. Your previous efforts to derive purpose in life by becoming a physician did not have the desired outcome. It has only made you prone to burnout while giving you a late start in life. Considering this result, you might feel reluctant to embark on such a search again.

The truth is that not developing and acting on a plan to improve your life will only exacerbate the duration and intensity of your emotional pain. The default response of learned helplessness does not provide any solutions to your current problems. It only creates the conditions for problems to intensify which sends you down a deeper spiral of depression, anxiety and burnout.

Have reasonable expectations of yourself when you pursue changes in your life. As type A, high-achieving perfectionists, we have a tendency of putting immense pressure on ourselves to accomplish too much too fast. Such pressure makes it more likely that you will freeze from high levels of anxiety or be discouraged if you do not immediately achieve the desired outcome. A healthier strategy is to approach this life-crafting exercise with curiosity and compassion. Be patient with yourself as you come up with realistic strategies to improve your life. Making incremental changes and sticking with them over a period of time can dramatically improve the quality of your life.

A good starting point is to employ a number of evidence-based tools discussed in this book to advocate for yourself. Embrace your leverage as a physician and set boundaries with parties that take advantage of your work ethic, compassion and altruism. Ask for longer time slots for patients with more complex medical histories. Refuse to take on additional work such as quality improvement and research projects that come with no additional compensation but financially penalize you due to reductions in clinical productivity. Advocating for such changes can help you find more fulfillment in clinical medicine by allowing you to focus on what matters most – providing the best possible patient care.

However, there are times when employers violate even the firmest of boundaries. You may be in a toxic situation where your efforts to advocate for yourself have reached a dead end. In such a situation, you need to explore your options. I have seen many physicians successfully navigate a career change both within and beyond clinical medicine.

Another reason to engage in a life-crafting exercise is because your sense of purpose can change over time. What was important to your younger self may not be as important to you today. Pressing pause to engage in self-reflection can protect you from the trap of automatically pursuing goals that are no longer aligned with your values. Evidence shows that we perform almost 50% of our actions with minimal conscious guidance (12).

As an example, professional achievement might have been important to you at an earlier stage of life. However, as you have grown older and wiser, you may not derive the same meaning from individual success. You may have discovered new sources of meaning such as spending quality time with loved ones or volunteering for a noble cause. In this scenario, you need to recalibrate your relationship with achievement to create the time and space to invest in your relationships or volunteering endeavors. The same holds true for your current job, which you might have found more appealing at an earlier phase of life. However, as you and your job have changed over time, it may be appropriate to assess how much it is contributing to your life satisfaction.

In his book *From Strength to Strength: Finding Success, Happiness and Deep Purpose in The Second Half of Life*, Arthur C. Brooks, a Harvard professor, describes how achievement-oriented individuals follow a predictable formula for success in their personal and professional lives: work tirelessly and make sacrifices to reach your goals. Though initially effective, this formula is not sustainable in the long run because your strengths and weaknesses evolve over time. As you get older, you lack the stamina or memory retention to maintain the same ferocious pace as your younger self. However, growing older comes with newfound strengths that result from having overcome a variety of life experiences. Such strengths include having more wisdom and the ability to enrich others through counsel. This dynamic process highlights the importance of assessing whether your career is aligned with your evolving traits (13).

However, you cannot solely rely on clinical medicine to fulfill your purpose in life. Medicine is only a part of who you are. You are more than a physician. You may forget this because clinical medicine has consumed a large portion of your waking hours. However, you are also likely a parent, spouse, partner, sibling, adult child, friend and community member. These intimate relationships are a valuable, though often underappreciated, source of purpose. Sacrificing these bonds at the altar of medicine will hurt you and the people who matter most to you.

Most importantly, you are a human being with unique strengths, abilities and interests. It is important to invest in yourself by exploring who you are outside clinical medicine. This process can lead to new insights and uncover skills that can help you be better equipped to handle the daily demands of clinical medicine.

As a personal example, engaging in the life-crafting exercise helped me realize that writing adds purpose to my life. This is a creative endeavor in which I play with words to articulate thoughts that hopefully provide pearls of wisdom to my readers. Writing is also a therapeutic exercise because it allows me to process thoughts and feelings about the challenges of practicing medicine. Furthermore, it serves as an impetus to review literature which sharpens my knowledge base.

However, you do not need to do something as dramatic as write a book to derive meaning. The act of being creative is meaningful in itself. During our work together, many physicians have shared examples of creative endeavors that helped them reduce burnout such as dust off a musical instrument, take a photography class, work on an art project, train to be a yoga instructor or read fiction books. A systematic review found that visual arts-based interventions can have positive effects on improving clinician burnout (14). In addition, creative writing outside of work can have a marked effect on improving overall well-being and even improve performance in the workplace (15). Such creative pursuits do not address the systemic factors interfering with your ability to care for patients. However, they can be a valuable source of purpose and meaning to help you better cope with the challenges of practicing clinical medicine.

Even hobbies can be a valuable source of purpose. I recently dusted off my childhood collection of baseball and football cards to share with my son. We have spent hours looking at them and talking about different athletes and their respective teams. Bringing these cards back to life has been a bonding experience that I will cherish for the rest of my life.

Being mindful of your inevitable death can be an important guide in your search for purpose. Let's return to Bronnie Ware's book which discusses the top five regrets of the dying. We discussed how systemic factors predispose you to the first regret which is not living a life true to yourself, but a life that meets the expectations of others. The remaining four regrets are:

1) "I wish I hadn't worked so hard."
2) "I wish I'd had the courage to express my feelings."

3) "I wish I had stayed in touch with my friends."
4) "I wish I had let myself be happier."

There is great despair when you realize that medicine predisposes you to every single regret. You worked tirelessly to become a physician and lost touch with countless friends along the way. The workload only continues after training as we often skip family and social events due to overnight, weekend and holiday responsibilities.

Medicine also interferes with your ability to express your feelings. As physicians, we often suffer in silence for fear of appearing weak or facing repercussions. We are also trained to be stoic in the face of suffering which we witness on a daily basis. Though useful in different clinical settings, stoicism can come at a cost to one's well-being. A study measuring the effects of stoic ideology across different cultures found it is negatively associated with subjective happiness and eudaimonic well-being (16). When you consistently dull your emotions, you don't only dampen difficult ones. You also end up with lower levels of happiness, joy and satisfaction.

Realizing that medicine predisposes you to every single regret of the dying may initially trigger feelings of despair. However, your newfound level of awareness is also a catalyst to take action and improve your life. You cannot overcome burnout and emotional difficulties by falling for the trap of learned helplessness. You will not find any meaning or purpose in a state of paralysis. You need to embark on a journey of self-reflection and make the necessary changes to extract more meaning from clinical medicine and beyond. This will spare you regrets on your death bed. *Memento mori*, remembering you must die, can be a powerful reminder to work on this essential antidote to burnout.

References

1. Viswanathan R. Death anxiety, locus of control and purpose in life of physicians: their relationship to patient death notification. *Psychosomatics.* 1996;37(4):339–345. https://doi.org/10.1016/S0033-3182(96)71546-3
2. Rainey L. The search for purpose in life: an exploration of purpose, the search process, and purpose anxiety. *University of Pennsylvania ScholarlyCommons.* Master of Applied Positive Psychology (MAPP) Capstone Projects. 60. August, 2014. https://core.ac.uk/reader/76383860
3. McKnight PE, Kashdan TB. Purpose in life as a system that creates and sustains health and well-being: an integrative, testable theory. *Review of General Psychology.* 2009;13(3):242–251. doi:10.1037/a0017152. https://cdn2.psychologytoday.com/assets/attachments/3382/mcknight-kashdan-2009-purpose-in-life-rev-gen-psy.pdf
4. Thoreau HD. *Walden.* Pan Macmillan. October, 2016.

5. Boreham ID, Schutte NS. The relationship between purpose in life and depression and anxiety: a meta-analysis. *J Clin Psychol*. 2023;79(12):2736–2767. doi:10.1002/jclp.23576

6. Sone T, Nakaya N, Ohmori K, et al. Sense of life worth living (ikigai) and mortality in Japan: Ohsaki Study. *Psychosom Med*. 2008;70(6):709–715. doi:10.1097/PSY.0b013e31817e7e64

7. Shanafelt TD, West CP, Sloan JA, et al. Career fit and burnout among academic faculty. *Arch Intern Med*. 2009;169(10):990–995. doi:10.1001/archinternmed.2009.70

8. Ware B. *Top five regrets of the dying: a life transformed by the dearly departed*. Hay House. August, 2019.

9. Maier SF, Seligman ME. Learned helplessness at fifty: insights from neuroscience. *Psychol Rev*. 2016;123(4):349–367. doi:10.1037/rev0000033

10. Schippers MC, Ziegler N. Life crafting as a way to find purpose and meaning in life. *Front Psychol*. 2019 Dec 13;10:2778. doi:10.3389/fpsyg.2019.02778

11. Schippers MC, Morisano D, Locke EA, et al. Writing about personal goals and plans regardless of goal type boosts academic performance. *Contemporary Educational Psychology*. 2020;60. Article 101823. https://doi.org/10.1016/j.cedpsych.2019.101823

12. Wood W, Quinn JM, Kashy DA. Habits in everyday life: thought, emotion and action. *Journal of Personality and Social Psychology*. December 2002;83(6):1281–1297. doi:10.1037/0022-3514.83.6.1281

13. Brooks AC. *From strength to strength: finding success, happiness and deep purpose in the second half of life*. Bloomsbury Publishing. 2022.

14. Engel T, Gowda D, Sandhu JS, Banerjee S. Art interventions to mitigate burnout in health care professionals: a systematic review. *Perm J*. 2023;27(2):184–194. doi:10.7812/TPP/23.018

15. Cronin M, Hubbard V, Cronin TA Jr, Frost P. Combatting professional burnout through creative writing. *Clin Dermatol*. 2020;38(5):512–515. doi:10.1016/j.clindermatol.2020.05.004

16. Karl JA, Verhaeghen P, Aikman SN, et al. Misunderstood stoicism: the negative association between stoic ideology and well-being. *J Happiness Stud*. 2022 Aug;23:3531–3547. https://doi.org/10.1007/s10902-022-00563-w

Part 4

A Path to a Better System

13 Promote Psychological Safety

The following scenario is familiar to anyone who has pursued a career in medicine. You go to the hospital early in the morning to round with your team on patients for the purpose of evaluating their condition and determining the next course of action. A team usually consists of an attending physician, a number of resident physicians and members from other disciplines such as pharmacy, nursing or social work.

At some point during the rounds, the attending physician puts a resident on the spot by asking them a series of questions about the case. This teaching tactic, known as pimping, is intended to gauge a resident's level of knowledge. Every detail of the case is fair game ranging from what was the patient's last set of vital signs to questions about the pharmacokinetics of their medications and potential drug interactions. Not answering questions correctly is often met with public displays of disapproval and criticism.

On the surface, this practice may seem like an efficient use of time. It makes sense for attending physicians to make the most of their time on rounds by assessing their residents' level of knowledge while they simultaneously provide patient care.

In reality, pimping is an ineffective teaching tactic that mistreats physicians-in-training and medical students. Instead of promoting learning, this tactic humiliates the learner by publicly displaying their lack of knowledge, further entrenching the power disparities engrained in medicine (1).

Go back to a moment in your training when your knowledge was put on display for everyone to judge. How did you feel after an attending employed this tactic on you? Did you feel good about yourself after the experience? Did you subsequently feel comfortable rounding with the same attending?

Odds are this experience had a negative impact on you. Perhaps you felt more anxious the next time you had to round with the same attending. You might have also felt timid to ask questions for fear of being judged as less competent. Such fear was not conducive to your

DOI: 10.4324/9781003473923-18

medical education because it shifted your focus from learning to self-preservation. You walked on eggshells for fear of being in such a vulnerable position.

The example of pimping highlights a fundamental problem plaguing medical culture – a lack of psychological safety. This concept refers to the amount of interpersonal risk one feels safe to take by sharing one's concerns or ideas, asking a question or admitting a lack of knowledge without the fear of retribution, negative judgment or being embarrassed. In a psychologically safe environment, team members are not afraid of being ostracized for expressing their perspectives. They respect each other's competence, have positive intentions towards one another, and are able to exchange constructive criticism (2).

Barriers to Psychological Safety

The tactic of pimping is only one barrier to psychological safety in medical culture. As discussed in chapter 4, medicine is plagued by bias, prejudice and discrimination based on someone's gender, ethnicity, race, religion, medical school of graduation, professional ranking and medical specialty. This can manifest in a variety of ways such as acts of microaggression which contribute to psychologically unsafe working and learning environments. Due to their subtle and covert nature, microaggressions can be difficult to detect and often go unnoticed, leaving the victim feeling isolated and dismissed (3).

Due to their covert nature, microaggressions tend to be recurrent which only prolongs their detrimental effects. A study of more than 7,400 surgical residents showed that nearly 50% of them had experienced at least one form of mistreatment, with 19.0% reporting exposure to mistreatment at least a few times per month and 30.9% reporting such exposure a few times per year (4).

It is essential to eradicate such behaviors, and their underlying attitudes, from medicine and society. They have a profound negative impact on mental health, making one vulnerable to depression, anxiety, imposter syndrome and burnout. They also disrupt the cohesion and morale of a healthcare organization (3).

Another factor eroding psychological safety is that, as physicians, we are not the best equipped in providing feedback to one another. I have encountered this in countless scenarios. As an example, an intern developed the habit of showing up a few minutes late to 7 am morning rounds. She did not believe being a few minutes tardy was a big deal because no senior resident or attending physician commented on her behavior. After all, she was already in the hospital tying some loose ends before morning rounds.

You and I both know how this situation plays out. The higher-ups on her treatment team silently stewed until they could no longer hide their feelings. Just prior to the end of the inpatient block, her chief resident screamed at her in front of the entire team for being unprofessional throughout the entire rotation. This aggressive tirade left the intern feeling confused and shocked because she had not received any prior indication that her behavior was upsetting anyone.

As a seasoned attending, I wish I had the opportunity to forewarn this intern that her behavior was going to get her in trouble. Showing up later than your higher-ups is frowned upon. If morning rounds are at 7 am, be prepared to show up early. Those lowest on the totem pole can expect to show up the earliest. The chief resident was justified in feeling frustrated by the intern's behaviors. However, he handled the situation poorly and unprofessionally. He should have never humiliated her in front of the entire team. Instead, he should have pulled her aside at the earliest sign of tardiness and educated her on the expectations for the rotation.

As another example, I worked with a physician in fellowship who during rounds asked the attending about their reasoning behind a chosen treatment modality. They prefaced the question by acknowledging they were unfamiliar with the treatment and hoping to learn. The attending responded by telling the fellow to read the chart to figure it out.

It is possible the fellow may have posed their question at an inopportune time. The attending may have felt pressed due to urgent clinical matters. However, their response was unprofessional and hurtful. They could have politely asked the fellow to table the conversation for a more opportune time. Instead, their dismissive comment created friction and dissuaded the fellow from asking further questions.

Such interactions illustrate how physicians engage with one another in ways that erode psychological safety. At times, we are our worst enemies and compound physician suffering by the way we treat each other.

Benefits of Psychological Safety

One of the primary benefits of psychological safety is the ability to speak up against injustice. Silence is associated with a lack of psychological safety (5). Due to a fear of potential repercussions, you are more likely to mind your own business rather than risk upsetting the medical establishment, even if it is for the greater good.

I worked with a resident who was struggling to keep up with the grueling call demands of her intern year. What helped her survive the heavy workload was staying focused on becoming a senior resident when she would no longer have to take call. As she approached the end of her intern year,

I asked her to consider whether it would have been beneficial if call had been more evenly distributed among all residents of the program. In other words, would she hypothetically be willing to take some call as a senior resident to alleviate some of the pressure off incoming interns? She was reluctant to support such a change in the call structure. She thought it was only fair that future incoming residents experienced the same brunt of call duties like her class did.

When you feel mistreated and taken advantage of, you are less likely to take action for the collective good. Your main objective is to find a way to survive rather than consider what is best for everyone involved. I am sure the intern felt it was not fair that her class carried the entire burden of call, while senior residents were completely exempt from it. Yet, she never felt safe to voice her perspective for fear of repercussions from senior residents. Instead, she suffered in silence until it was her turn to perpetuate the unloading of burdens on subordinates.

This pattern of behavior is not limited to residents. As another example, I worked with a hospitalist who dreaded going into work. He felt tremendous anxiety the night prior to his shifts. He described feeling overwhelmed by the workload. He was often responsible for over 20 patients per day, many of whom were seriously ill and spread throughout different floors of the hospital. Any requests for relief such as putting a cap on the number of patients he was responsible for or being assigned patients in close physical proximity fell on the deaf ears of leadership. Nor was there any extra compensation for carrying a larger number of patients or signing up for extra shifts.

Due to the grueling workload, their group was short-staffed and had a hard time recruiting new hospitalists. Yet, hospitalists within the group were reluctant to chip in and help each other out. In his words, "Why would I volunteer to take on an extra shift if it is going to come at a cost to my mental and physical health due to getting slammed at work?"

As another example, an early career attending joined an established practice consisting of senior attendings. She was immediately responsible for taking on all new patient referrals and same day urgent appointments for all established patients. It was only a matter of time before this disproportionate allocation of work led to her burnout. During one of our sessions, we explored how the lack of psychological safety prevented her from speaking to her colleagues about the situation.

Staying silent is understandable when you don't feel safe. This is an act of self-preservation. However, this approach only makes you more vulnerable to exploitation. It also erodes team morale by perpetuating acts of injustice and mistreatment across an organization. Cultivating psychological safety is a powerful antidote against mistreatment stemming from bias and discrimination. It is essential for individuals with lower ranking in the medical hierarchy to feel safe to speak up in order to eradicate bias and discrimination from medicine.

We cannot be complicit in silence. It is the responsibility of every physician, especially those in positions of authority, to speak up against bias and discrimination. Otherwise, they will continue to plague medicine. Shedding a light on them and their negative impact is the only way to eliminate them.

An additional benefit of psychological safety is that it promotes a healthier learning environment. You are more likely to ask questions if you are not afraid of being judged as less competent. You are also more open to questions assessing your clinical knowledge and feedback on your clinical performance if you believe their intention is to make you a better physician rather than disparage you. A study of physicians at an academic medical center showed that physicians with higher levels of psychological safety were more open to receiving corrective performance feedback and suggestions for improvement (6).

Psychological safety also promotes help-seeking behavior. A survey of surgical resident and attending physicians showed the vast majority (94%) anticipated wanting support for a stressful situation in the future such as an adverse patient outcome or involvement in a legal situation. In addition, the majority of respondents had been involved in a serious adverse patient event (53%) or had experienced a personal stressor (57%) in the past year. Despite the prevalence of stressful experiences in one's personal and professional life, 68% of respondents would not seek help due to concerns about a potential negative impact on their career (7).

Asking for help and support requires you to be vulnerable. You need to put your guard down to be seen, heard and understood. This is the only way someone can truly understand what you are going through and provide you with individualized help specific to your situation. Without such vulnerability, the best they can do is offer generic advice that may or may not be applicable to you. It is the cultivation of psychological safety that allows for help-seeking behavior to occur.

Furthermore, psychological safety enhances physician wellness by serving as a powerful antidote to burnout. A cross-sectional analysis of survey data from 715 small-to-medium-size U.S. primary care practices found that practices in which no members reported burnout had higher levels of psychological safety. According to this study, practices with zero burnout also reported higher levels of adaptive reserve, the use of quality improvement strategies, being clinician-owned and lower rates of participation in accountable care organizations (8).

Most importantly, psychological safety enhances patient care. A psychologically safe environment encourages self-assessment, engagement in quality improvement and the opportunity for staff to speak up about potential errors (9). Such practices facilitate the exchange of information in medicine which is a complex, dynamic and high stakes work environment.

How to Increase Psychological Safety

Organizational interventions spearheaded by leadership are essential to promote psychological safety within every healthcare setting. They need to establish clear and concise policies to promote safety and prevent misuse of power. Penalties should be imposed on those who abuse their leverage. More women and members of minority groups need to be hired in leadership positions to reflect the growing diversity of the physician workforce. Those in leadership should be visible and open to feedback from members of the healthcare organization.

Systemic interventions are necessary but not sufficient. The responsibility of promoting a culture of psychological safety cannot fall solely on the system. Each one of us plays an important role in promoting psychological safety within our environments based on how we interact with others.

Lead by example by treating everyone with respect regardless of their role on the team. Be appreciative of the pivotal role that advanced practice providers, nurses, psychologists, social workers and office staff play in patient care. We cannot serve our patients without their help.

Use the Socratic method when you pose questions to residents and medical students. Unlike the teaching tactic of pimping, the Socratic method asks questions in a methodical manner with the intent of helping the learner make new connections in their body of knowledge and enhance their critical thinking skills. Instead of posing questions in rapid succession, incorporate pauses to allow the learner to think before they reflexively respond (10). If the trainee does not know an answer, give them grace. Do not humiliate them but reframe their lack of knowledge as a learning opportunity. After all, medicine is a constantly evolving field and lifelong learning is essential to practicing medicine. The purpose of any teaching session should be to normalize the pursuit of knowledge.

If you see a change in a colleague's behavior, such as an increase in irritability, showing up to work late, being unkempt or quieter than usual, check on them. Ask them how they are doing and hold space for their answer. Make yourself available should they want to reach out in the future.

Be proactive and constructive when offering feedback. The start of a new rotation can be challenging for residents as they try to decipher and adapt to new expectations. Be clear about what you expect from them at the very onset of the rotation. Remember that residents change rotations every four weeks. Every transition comes with new roles, expectations, clinical responsibilities and team dynamics. Be patient as this transition can be difficult.

Let go of perfectionism. This is not an invitation to complacency or substandard work. On the contrary, it is the recognition that to err is to be human. You cannot have a good clinical outcome every single time. Projecting such unrealistic expectations intimidates early career physicians and those in training. It also sets them up for failure. Acknowledging our vulnerability to mistakes allows us to be more vigilant of them. The ability to have open conversations when mistakes occur and examine them with curiosity is essential to learn from them. This is not consistent with a perfectionist mindset which implies there is no further room for personal growth. This is a dangerous mindset which hinders self-examination by creating a false illusion that we are immune to error.

Substitute the competitive mindset for a collaborative approach. Being competitive was engrained in you during your journey to become a physician. You competed against peers to get into a prestigious college, medical school and residency of choice. As an attending, you need to let go of this mindset. What served you in the past no longer serves you today. You are more likely to excel in medicine by working in synergy with colleagues who have different areas of expertise than you. The amount of information is too vast for any single physician to master.

Changing your mindset and way of communicating will enhance the psychological safety and morale within your team. More importantly, such changes will have a profound long-term impact on the culture of medicine. You are providing a blueprint to positively influence the way future attending physicians think, act and communicate with one another.

One of the best parts of treating physicians is hearing stories of how they support one another. It gives me hope that medicine will evolve into a more humane and compassionate profession when physicians share heartwarming examples of promoting psychological safety and cohesion.

An attending described holding coffee rounds with residents and medical students. During these rounds, the attending would check in on them while they enjoyed a cup of coffee. As another example, a fellow described reaching out to incoming fellows to welcome them to the program and ask if they needed any help with the transition. A senior resident described the habit of reaching out to interns after working with them on a rotation to see how they were doing and ask how the rotation could improve.

Such examples tell me that despite the numerous challenges plaguing medicine, there are also many kind and caring physicians who will help medicine evolve into a more compassionate and collaborative profession that embraces the humanity in every single one of us.

References

1. Kost A, Chen FM. Socrates was not a pimp: changing the paradigm of questioning in medical education. *Acad Med*. 2015;90(1):20–24. doi:10.1097/ACM.0000000000000446
2. Edmonsdon A. Psychological safety and learning behavior in work teams. *Administrative Science Quarterly*. 1999;44(2):350–383. https://doi.org/10.2307/2666999
3. Desai V, Conte AH, Nguyen VT, et al. Veiled harm: impacts of microaggressions on psychological safety and physician burnout. *Perm J*. 2023;27(2):169–178. doi:10.7812/TPP/23.017
4. Hu YY, Ellis RJ, Hewitt DB, et al. Discrimination, abuse, harassment, and burnout in surgical residency training. *N Engl J Med*. 2019;381(18):1741–1752. doi:10.1056/NEJMsa1903759
5. Brinsfield CT. Employee silence motives: investigation of dimensionality and development of measures. *J Organ Behav*. 2013;34(5):671–697. doi:10.1002/job.1829
6. Scheepers RA, van den Goor M, Arah OA, Heineman MJ, Lombarts KMJMH. Physicians' perceptions of psychological safety and peer performance feedback. *J Contin Educ Health Prof*. 2018;38(4):250–254. doi:10.1097/CEH.0000000000000225
7. Hu YY, Fix ML, Hevelone ND, et al. Physicians' needs in coping with emotional stressors: the case for peer support. *Arch Surg*. 2012;147(3):212–217. doi:10.1001/archsurg.2011.312
8. Edwards ST, Marino M, Solberg LI, et al. Cultural and structural features of zero-burnout primary care practices. *Health Aff (Millwood)*. 2021;40(6):928–936. doi:10.1377/hlthaff.2020.02391
9. O'Donovan R, McAuliffe E. A systematic review exploring the content and outcomes of interventions to improve psychological safety, speaking up and voice behaviour. *BMC Health Serv Res*. 2020 Feb 10;20(1):101. doi:10.1186/s12913-020-4931-2
10. Stoddard HA, O'Dell DV. Would Socrates have actually used the "Socratic method" for clinical teaching? *J Gen Intern Med*. 2016;31(9):1092–1096. doi:10.1007/s11606-016-3722-2

14 Invest in Physician Wellness

Many hospitals are experiencing financial challenges that have been exacerbated by the aftermaths of the COVID pandemic and the rising cost of labor and medical supplies. According to healthcare consulting practice leaders, hospitals are under tremendous financial pressure because revenue is not keeping up with inflation (1). In response to this reality, it is understandable that hospitals would look for ways to reduce expenditures and generate additional revenue. On the surface, investing in physician wellness does not appear to be aligned with these financial goals.

The truth is that prioritizing physician wellness is a sound financial and strategic decision because burnout comes at a great cost to hospitals. National surveys indicate that burnout puts physicians at risk of reducing their clinical work hours and leaving practice (2, 3). This is a serious threat to hospitals, many of which are already short-staffed. According to a cross-sectional study of 18,719 academic physicians, 32.6% of participants had a moderate or higher intent to leave within two years (3). Institutions that fail to address the burnout epidemic are vulnerable to staff shortages that could interfere with their ability to provide vital clinical services to their patient population.

In addition, burnout can negatively impact the operating budget of any hospital due to an overall reduction in clinical productivity. On a national scale, it is estimated that the cost associated with physician turnover and reduced clinical hours due to burnout is approximately $4.6 billion each year (4). A cross-sectional analysis found that turnover of primary care physicians (PCP) results in approximately $979 million in excess healthcare expenditures, with $260 million attributed to PCP burnout-related turnover (5).

On an organizational level, hospitals lose significant revenue when physicians leave. It is estimated that physicians generate on average $2.4 million each year, with some specialists generating up to $3.48 million per year (6). The financial hit is exacerbated by the delay in recruiting new

DOI: 10.4324/9781003473923-19

physicians to replace departed ones. It takes about 4.3 months to replace a family physician and 5–10 months to replace a medical or surgical specialist (7). Of note, these estimates do not take into account the time it takes for incoming physicians to build their caseloads and reach the same level of productivity as their departed counterparts.

As a case example, Stanford University studied physician turnover attributable to self-reported burnout and the associated financial burden. They found that physicians who reported burnout had an 168% increased likelihood of leaving their institution within two years. It is worth noting that factors such as depression, anxiety, work hours and surgical specialty were not statistically significant predictors of physician turnover. They also calculated the cost of physician recruitment to range between $268,000 and $957,000 per physician based on specialty, years of experience and expertise. The cumulative two-year economic loss due to physician departure attributable to burnout was estimated between $15,544,000 and $55,506,000 (8).

These staggering numbers make it abundantly clear that hospitals do not have a financial choice but to invest in physician wellness. Trying to avoid the expenses associated with combating physician burnout is the equivalent of adopting a penny-wise, but pound-foolish mentality because the cumulative cost of burnout is too great to ignore. Organizational interventions aimed at promoting physician well-being can improve job performance and reduce the likelihood that physicians will leave their current practice. A randomized clinical trial of 74 practicing physicians at the Mayo Clinic showed that physicians who were offered paid protected time to participate in facilitated discussion groups experienced increased work engagement and the improvement was sustained 12 months following the intervention (9). Such outcomes highlight how investments in physician wellness are a long-term benefit for both physicians and employers.

However, there is another strategic reason for hospitals to invest in physician wellness. The imminent physician shortage will make it even harder and more expensive for hospitals to recruit and retain physicians. According to the National Center for Health Workforce Analysis, there is an overall projected shortage of 81,180 full-time equivalent physicians by 2035 assuming current patterns of attrition, work participation and graduation (10). This trend will only force remaining physicians to *carry an even heavier workload in the future, which will make them more vulnerable to burnout and career dissatisfaction.*

Hospitals may choose to circumvent this shortage by increasingly relying on nurse practitioners and physician assistants for certain services. This is a short-cut solution that does not address the root of the problem. Though they are an essential part of the healthcare system, advanced practice providers do not have the same medical training and qualifications as physicians. As the population continues to age and have more complex medical needs, hospitals will face increased pressure to employ physicians for essential clinical services. Hospitals which prioritize and invest in physician wellness will have a competitive advantage over those that fail to address the systemic factors contributing to burnout in their institutions.

The reasons to invest in physician wellness extend beyond the financial realm. There is an ethical responsibility to make it a priority. Physicians make tremendous sacrifices to complete their medical training and work tirelessly to provide patient care. Yet, practicing clinical medicine jeopardizes their mental health. Hospitals cannot wash their hands clean of their role in the current predicament and put the entire onus of combating burnout on physicians. Not taking any action to address the problem is the equivalent of saying that physicians are solely responsible for their suffering. Not only is this perspective not accurate, it is also a form of gaslighting that completely absolves responsible parties by blaming those impacted by systemic factors.

Burnout cannot be eradicated without organizational engagement and a commitment to making the necessary systemic changes that improve clinical medicine. A meta-analysis of 19 studies found that organization-driven interventions targeting the work environment had stronger effects compared to individual-focused interventions (11). Organizations need to acknowledge how they have contributed to the problem and work together with physicians to eradicate it.

Healthcare should be the embodiment of kindness and compassion. It should be an environment where everyone feels cared for, respected and valued. Treating healthcare workers like a cog in a wheel whose sole purpose is to generate revenue is a dehumanizing process that is not congruent with the essence of medicine. As physicians, we push our feelings to the side and show up to care for our patients. Even during the most treacherous times, such as the COVID pandemic when there was a shortage of protective equipment, you can count on physicians to show up, often risking their lives, because it is the right thing to do. We have taken an oath to help the sick and honor it at all times. It is not much to ask hospitals to also do the right thing and address the systemic factors contributing to burnout. However, if ethical reasons are not aligned with business practices and balancing operating budgets, then I hope the financial arguments in this chapter will incentivize hospitals to prioritize physician wellness in their institutions.

Reason for Hope

On a positive note, physician wellness is coming to the national forefront as an urgent issue that requires immediate attention. The United

States Surgeon General, Dr. Vivek Murthy, issued an advisory highlighting the urgent need to address the healthcare worker burnout crisis across the country (12). In addition, Congress passed the Dr. Lorna Breen Act to bolster the mental health infrastructure that supports physicians and other healthcare providers. Furthermore, the Accreditation Council of Graduate Medical Education has incorporated resident physician wellness into its Common Program Requirements for all accredited residency and fellowship programs (13).

Hospitals cannot ignore these trends. A good starting point is for hospitals to invest in a robust wellness program which offers a variety of services such as free and confidential access to psychotherapy, psychiatric services and peer support groups. Such a program should also offer a curriculum on wellness education, interpersonal communication skills, conflict management and personal development. The good news is that different institutions are creating such wellness programs. Examples include the Stanford Medicine WellMD and WellPhD Center, the Mayo Clinic Program on Physician Well-Being, the Oregon Health and Science University Resident and Faculty Wellness Program, the UC Davis Clinician Health and Well-being Program and the University of Michigan Office of Well-Being.

On a more personal note, I have the privilege of serving physicians through the Akron Physician Wellness Initiative (APWI). The birth of this program was spearheaded by Dr. Joseph Varley, Chair of the Summa Health Department of Psychiatry, and Dr. Rob McGregor, former Chief Medical Officer at Akron Children's Hospital.

APWI offers physicians and advanced practice practitioners 12 free appointments per calendar year. Our clinical team includes three full-time psychologists and a 0.5 full-time equivalent psychiatrist. Services include wellness education, psychotherapy and psychiatric services. We also offer incoming residents a wellness check-in as an opportunity to have a safe and confidential conversation with a mental health provider about how things are going in their personal and professional lives. We have been operating since 2021 and have had the privilege of serving hundreds of healthcare providers. Health insurance is not utilized because the program is free of cost. To further promote confidentiality, we do not use an electronic medical record and only document in paper charts. Appointments can take place in person or via telehealth, based on provider preference.

One of the goals of this program has been to reduce barriers that prevent healthcare providers from seeking mental healthcare. 47.5% of providers who received services from APWI reported that they would not have sought any mental healthcare if it weren't for this program (14). This result shows that programs genuinely invested in physician wellness can reduce the stigma associated with seeking mental health and promote a culture which normalizes the pursuit of such care.

At the American Psychiatric Association Annual Conference in 2022, we shared testimonials from healthcare providers who received services at APWI. Here is what they said (15):

> "This experience has been so beyond helpful for me. I am so glad that I took advantage of this program as I was very hesitant to go to any sort of counseling. I feel like I'm getting my life back! Thank you to all who make this program possible."

> "Seeing [provider] on a consistent basis has become an essential part of my lifestyle. Being able to talk through difficult situations at work has made me a better physician and colleague, and had immeasurable benefits for my overall health."

> "I don't think words can fully express the magnitude of how much APWI has changed my life for the better. Being a physician, we see a lot of things throughout our days at work. However, outside of work we are people with human problems."

These testimonials highlight the impact that a robust wellness program has on combating burnout, promoting individual well-being and enhancing morale within an organization. However, such a program alone is not sufficient because burnout is a multifaceted problem that requires a comprehensive approach to address it. A variety of organizational interventions are necessary to eradicate burnout. Additional actions that hospitals can take include:

- Regularly monitor physician well-being by using validated instruments to proactively support staff with higher burnout scores.
- Invest in physicians' professional, educational and leadership development through generous CME stipends, paid time off and conference sponsorships.
- Align providers with work they find clinically meaningful.
- Hire sufficient support staff to reduce the administrative and clerical burden on physicians.
- Create comfortable communal spaces which allow staff to come together.
- Implement organizational strategies that promote diversity and inclusion, and eradicate different forms of bias.
- Give physicians more control of their work schedules and the autonomy to best determine the proper time allotment for patient encounters.

- Allocate time in the workday to allow physicians to complete required documentation and administrative tasks.
- Advance gender equity by eradicating pay inequality.
- Provide generous paid parental leave.
- Adopt policies to support women who carry a greater share of care-giving responsibilities.
- Facilitate physician engagement in physical activity by creating exercise rooms within hospital premises or sponsoring gym memberships.
- Provide staff with healthy food options at the cafeteria.
- Allow greater work flexibility including remote work when possible.
- Appoint a chief wellness officer who can direct the coordination and implementation of different interventions to promote physician wellness.

It is also important for hospitals to abandon a mindset that expects maximal clinical productivity from physicians. Such a tactic may maximize revenue in a given year. However, it is a myopic approach that ultimately backfires. Pushing healthcare providers to their limits by trying to squeeze every ounce of productivity out of them is a recipe for discontent and disgruntlement in the workplace. Physicians may endure such demands for a brief period of time, but will ultimately succumb to the physical, mental and social consequences of burnout. In a desperate attempt to survive, they cut back on their clinical hours or leave their job which places further pressures on the hospital to make up for the departures. The reflex is to squeeze even more work out of the remaining healthcare providers, which only exacerbates the problem. It is the equivalent of blowing air on a spreading fire, without addressing the fundamental problem and its myriad of consequences.

A healthier approach is to adopt a mindset of sustainable productivity. The goal of such a tactic is to keep physicians productive at reasonable levels without compromising their physical, mental or social health. This approach requires transparency from hospital administrators and physician engagement. Physicians should be included in determining productivity benchmarks and how to reach them.

Hospital administration may initially be reluctant to adopt such an approach because of concerns that it may not be the most profitable for the organization in a given year. However, such fears are unfounded because physicians are hard-working, altruistic perfectionists who are intrinsically motivated to maintain high levels of productivity. In addition, this approach does not come with the same pitfalls as trying to maximize physician prod-uctivity. By giving healthcare providers more breathing room, hospitals protect themselves from the financial impact of higher physician turnover and lower engagement.

More importantly, adopting a more sustainable approach to productivity improves morale among staff because they feel valued, respected and truly cared for. Promoting a healthy work culture improves not only retainment but also recruitment of future physicians.

To embrace this new strategy, hospitals need to conceptualize physicians differently. We are more than a line item on a financial spreadsheet and our worth goes beyond how much money we generate for a hospital system. We are human beings who care about making a positive impact in the lives of our patients. We suffer because of the countless administrative barriers that prevent us from delivering care to the best of our ability and need the help of hospital leadership to overcome these barriers. Let's work together to make medicine more efficient, effective and humane. Such a radical change will benefit hospitals, physicians and, most importantly, patients.

References

1. Morse S. Cash shortages plague hospitals but there are signs of improvement ahead. *Healthcare Finance*. July 7, 2023. Accessed February 23, 2024. https://www.healthcarefinancenews.com/news/cash-shortages-plague-hospitals#:~:text=Many%20hospitals%20are%20facing%20a,their%20financial%20covenants%20with%20lenders
2. Sinsky CA, Dyrbye LN, West CP, Satele D, Tutty M, Shanafelt TD. Professional satisfaction and the career plans of US physicians. *Mayo Clin Proc*. 2017;92(11):1625–1635. doi:10.1016/j.mayocp.2017.08.017
3. Ligibel JA, Goularte N, Berliner JI, et al. Well-being parameters and intention to leave current institution among academic physicians. *JAMA Netw Open*. 2023;6(12):e2347894. doi:10.1001/jamanetworkopen.2023.47894
4. Han S, Shanafelt TD, Sinsky CA, et al. Estimating the attributable cost of physician burnout in the United States. *Ann Intern Med*. 2019;170(11):784–790. doi:10.7326/M18-1422.
5. Sinsky CA, Shanafelt TD, Dyrbye LN, Sabety AH, Carlasare LE, West CP. Health care expenditures attributable to primary care physician overall and burnout-related turnover: a cross-sectional analysis. *Mayo Clin Proc*. 2022;97(4):693–702. doi:10.1016/j.mayocp.2021.09.013
6. Dyrda L. The cost of physician turnover. *Becker's Hospital CFO Report*. September 21, 2023. Accessed February 23, 2024. https://www.beckershospitalreview.com/finance/the-cost-of-physician-turnover.html
7. Stajduhar, T. The high costs of hiring the wrong physician. *NEJM CareerCenter*. Accessed February 23, 2024. https://www.nejmcareercenter.org/minisites/rpt/the-high-costs-of-hiring-the-wrong-physician/
8. Hamidi MS, Bohman B, Sandborg C, et al. Estimating institutional physician turnover attributable to self-reported burnout and associated financial burden: a case study. *BMC Health Serv Res*. 2018 Nov 27;18(1):851. doi:10.1186/s12913-018-3663-z
9. West CP, Dyrbye LN, Rabatin JT, et al. Intervention to promote physician well-being, job satisfaction, and professionalism: a randomized clinical trial. *JAMA Intern Med*. 2014;174(4):527–533. doi:10.1001/jamainternmed.2013.14387

10. National Center for Health Workforce Analysis. Physician workforce: projections, 2020-2035. November 2022. Accessed February 24, 2024. https://bhw.hrsa.gov/sites/default/files/bureau-health-workforce/Physicians-Projections-Factsheet.pdf
11. Panagioti M, Panagopoulou E, Bower P, et al. Controlled interventions to reduce burnout in physicians: a systematic review and meta-analysis. *JAMA Intern Med*. 2017;177(2):195–205. doi:10.1001/jamainternmed.2016.7674
12. Murthy V.H. Addressing health worker burnout, the U.S. Surgeon General's advisory on building a thriving health workforce. 2022. Accessed March 2, 2024. https://www.hhs.gov/sites/default/files/health-worker-wellbeing-advisory.pdf
13. Accreditation Council for Graduate Medical Education. Improving physician well-being, restoring meaning in medicine. Accessed March 1, 2024. https://www.acgme.org/meetings-and-educational-activities/physician-well-being/
14. Akron Physician Wellness Initiative. Empowering physicians in care. Accessed February 24, 2024. https://www.akronphysicianwellness.org/services
15. Varley J, Tsatiris D, Rowan C, Miller ANR. From innovation to collaboration: how two local hospitals are working together to provide physicians access to barrier-free mental healthcare. Conference Presentation at the American Psychiatric Association Annual Convention. May 2023. San Francisco, California, United States.

Index